Decolonization of Psychiatry in Jamaica

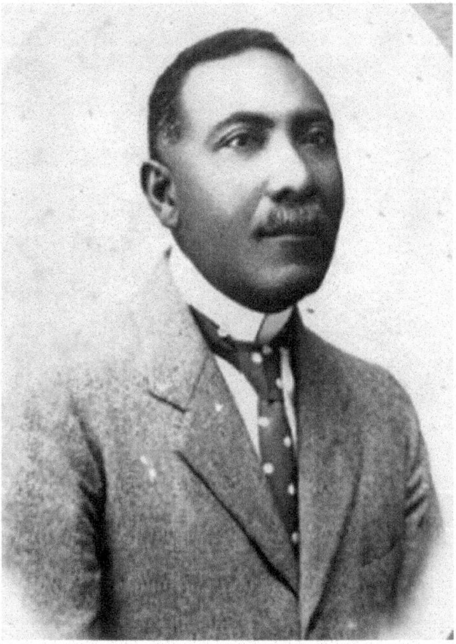

Dr. Hopetoun Edward Bond, MD, CM (Queen's University Canada); LRCP, LRCS (Edinburgh and Glasgow); Diploma in Psychological Medicine (Canada); Acting Senior Medical Officer, Jamaica Lunatic Asylum, August 1915–1919. *The first Black psychiatrist in the Caribbean.*

Frederick W. Hickling

Decolonization of Psychiatry in Jamaica

Madnificent Irations

palgrave
macmillan

Frederick W. Hickling
Department of Psychology
University of the West Indies
Kingston, Jamaica

ISBN 978-3-030-48488-0 ISBN 978-3-030-48489-7 (eBook)
https://doi.org/10.1007/978-3-030-48489-7

Cover illustration: Maram_shutterstock.com

This Palgrave Macmillan imprint is published by the registered company Springer Nature Switzerland AG
The registered company address is: Gewerbestrasse 11, 6330 Cham, Switzerland

Dedicated to Granduncle Hopetoun Edward Bond 1879–1939,
the first Black psychiatrist in the Caribbean

Publisher's Note

It was with profound sadness that we learned that Professor Hickling had died while this book was in production. In accordance with the wishes of his widow Hilary Hickling, copy editing was undertaken and reviewed by the publisher. We have worked to ensure that, as far as possible, the published text reflects the author's voice and intentions.

Contents

List of Figures

CHAPTER 1

Introduction

The system left by Westminster
has one intrinsic flaw
It forces us to divide and fight sisters
and brothers with tooth and nail and claw. [1]

As a psychiatrist of nearly fifty years' experience, British psychiatry has been seminally involved in every phase of my professional development and practice. My mother tongue is English, and my worldview is Anglophone. I was born and raised in Jamaica, the miscegenated descendant of an ex-slave (my great-grandmother) and an English slave owner (my great-grandfather). I have been practicing psychiatry in the Caribbean since 1970. My work has been mainly in Jamaica, but I have had clinical experience in other Anglophone Caribbean territories, in New Zealand, and in England. During the course of my professional career I have encountered thousands of Caribbean people, descendants of Africans enslaved in the New World. I have also examined and treated migrants resident in England and the Caribbean, Europeans both in their home countries and when abroad, and, during a stay lasting six months, Europeans and Maoris in New Zealand. I worked for nearly five years of my senior professional life as a consultant psychiatrist in Birmingham and the Midlands, between 1995 and 2000, as one of four Black consultant psychiatrists in Britain at that time. Although I have lived and worked for most of my career in Jamaica, I was trained mainly by British psychiatrists and/or British trained psychiatrists. Significant swathes of my medical

F. W. Hickling, *Decolonization of Psychiatry in Jamaica*,
https://doi.org/10.1007/978-3-030-48489-7_1

and psychiatric training occurred in the UK, but most of my medical training and experience has been in Jamaica and the Caribbean.

Between the passage of the Emancipation Act in 1833 and the attainment of full freedom (the end of apprenticeship) in 1838, the notion of educating the African slaves encountered strong opposition from plantation and slave owners, despite the efforts of many Christian missionaries seeking to provide religious education as a means of converting the Africans to Christianity [2]. The majority of the White population, who could afford it, sent their sons to be educated in England as 'there was no equivalent of a good English grammar school education to be had in the West Indies' [3]. The demand for classical secondary and higher education during and after the mid-1800s was bolstered by economic decline due to weakened sugar revenues, growth of the local middle class, and the increased availability of lower level white-collar jobs to non-Whites [4]. During the latter half of the nineteenth century, a number of secondary schools were established across the British West Indies. In Jamaica, one of the early secondary schools was Wolmer's High School in Kingston, established in 1729 (https://www.wolmersboyshigh.org/history). Wolmer's High School is a case study of an important institution devised by colonial British society, designed to shape the hegemonic control of colonies like Jamaica. John Wolmer, a wealthy goldsmith, bequeathed the bulk of his estate for the foundation of a free school in the parish where he died. A resolution of the school's trustees of September 15, 1777 restricted admission to Whites only [5]. By 1815, the school started to admit pupils of color. By the end of the nineteenth century, a select group of entirely Black pupils attained admission to this school. Among that select group were my grandfather Frederick Pape Bond, his elder brother Hopetoun Edward Bond, and their brothers and sisters. They were among the first Blacks in Jamaica at that time to receive a coveted high school education. It was a period shortly after the Emancipation Act came into force in 1834, when the British colonial government was just beginning to open educational facilities to Black people. In fact it was a period when Whites worldwide were just beginning to allow token Black representatives to enter secondary and tertiary level institutions.

Few people who have not actually experienced an English colonial society can really understand the effect of colonialism on young minds. Many of us were Brown-skinned, as equally distinguishable from our Black African brothers as from our White English cousins and half brothers and sisters. As privileged middle-class school children, we were exposed to a form of socialization and education modeled on the blueprints of the British public school system. Counter to what is usually implied by 'public', these schools were, by the nineteenth century, socially exclusive, private institutions, designed to shape the minds of the youth of the British ruling class. The assimilation of the British business classes to the social pattern of the gentry and aristocracy proceeded rapidly from the early nineteenth century onwards. In 1869, they were more or less set free from all government control and set about elaborating that actively anti-intellectual, anti-scientific, games-dominated Tory imperialism which was to remain characteristic of them [6]. The public school was the factory designed to perpetuate the gene pool repository of the European delusion that Whites were born to rule the world by divine right. Imagine the experience we had, as Brown cousins, descendants of Black Africans enslaved in the New World and miscegenated children of our White rulers, growing together in schools that taught us Latin and Greek, fine arts, the classics, European history and the humanities, together with mathematics, calculus, and the sciences. Our parallel exposure to cricket and other British sports and to the Army and Air Cadet Force was designed to shape our future as agents of British Imperialism in the colonies. Our teachers were predominantly Brown- and Black-skinned Jamaicans with similar educational backgrounds, although our senior teachers, headmasters, and headmistresses were usually White British. We were being taught to be agents of the European psychosis [7] in Brown and Black skins.

My granduncle Hopetoun Edward Bond (1879–1939), from Wolmer's High School for Boys in Kingston, won a scholarship to study medicine at Queen's University in Canada and became one of the first Blacks to graduate as a medical doctor from that institution in the early twentieth century. He also qualified as a Licentiate of the Royal College of Physicians and Surgeons of Edinburgh and of Glasgow. While my grandfather Frederick Pape was climbing the ranks of the Jamaican Civil Service as an accountant, Hopetoun qualified as a psychiatrist. He was awarded the Diploma in Psychological Medicine (Canada), one of the first Black graduates to obtain that degree and the first to originate from the Caribbean. He was also a member of the British Medical Association, engaging in private practice in Glasgow, where, during the course of 1910–1911, he was assistant and locum tenens to a Dr. Murison.

Black Jamaican psychiatrists are a rare breed. There was only a mere dozen or so of us in the world at the end of the twentieth century. The fact that the first known Black Jamaican and Caribbean psychiatrist, Hopetoun Bond, was my granduncle makes my presence in this group an even greater privilege, and perhaps not a coincidence in the overall scheme of things. My ontogeny represents a mongrel mixture of African and European miscegenation and is an important pivotal point for the discussion that follows. The African and European miscegenation in Jamaica and the Caribbean presents a unique natural selection process of the European colonial experience.

In 1911 Hopetoun returned to Jamaica to work in private practice in Kingston; in October 1914 he was appointed Junior Medical Officer at the Jamaica Lunatic Asylum (later the Bellevue Hospital), as a temporary replacement for Dr. Thomas Francis Shackleton, who was away on war service. Hopetoun was both a clinician and a medical academic, having authored 'Causation and Treatment of Pellagra,' published in 1915 in the London-based *Journal of Tropical Medicine and Hygiene* and New York-based *Medical Record*; three years later 'A Case of Porencephaly' appeared in the *British Medical Journal.* In August 1916 he was appointed Acting Physician Superintendent at the asylum [8]. He was not confirmed in the post, as it was the policy of the British colonial government not to appoint Blacks to top leadership positions in the Civil Service. The personnel pressures of World War I dictated that appropriate White professionals who would normally fill such posts were siphoned off from the Colonial Service to serve in the European theatre of war. Appointment to 'acting' or non-confirmed positions was a common practice in the administrative personnel hierarchy of the British Civil Service as a means of manipulation and of control of managers and employees. It was a manipulative maneuver, a ploy used by the Colonial Service, especially during crisis periods like the two World Wars, to fill the job positions of senior colonial civil servants with qualified native workers in temporary or acting positions. Once the crisis was over, the colonial job would be returned to a White civil servant and the acting native worker would be displaced and returned to a lesser position. This is an example of one of the administrative tools developed within the context of the European psychosis, for the maintenance of racial social control.

At the end of hostilities, Hopetoun tasted the bitter racism of this British Colonial administrative maneuver when he was removed from the position of Acting Physician Superintendent and replaced by a young English doctor returning from the front who was considerably junior to himself. In his rage, responding to what he regarded as a dose of virulent colonial racism, granduncle Hopetoun stormed out of the asylum, the Physician Superintendent job and Jamaica. Paradoxically, he returned to the UK where he had been trained as a medical practitioner and set up in private practice in London. He was especially angry, as the young man who replaced him in the top job at the mental hospital did not even have psychiatric qualifications. Hopetoun died in obscurity in London in 1939, a victim of the English variety of the European psychosis. It was acceptable at the time to educate a few Black people and even to allow them into the system, but under no circumstance was power to be shared with them. The tradition of White doctors running and controlling the Jamaica Lunatic Asylum continued until the mid-1930s, when another Black Jamaican, Roy Olivier Cooke (appointed OBE in 1964), a psychiatrist trained at Dalhousie University, Canada, was recruited by this institution and became its second Black Senior Medical Officer. He was followed in that post by Jamaicans Dr. Kenneth Royes, and (post independence) by Dr. Vincent O. Williams.

Fast-forward sixty years from granduncle Hopetoun's period as Acting SMO. My colleague Dr. Trevor Lindsay was appointed Acting SMO at Bellevue Hospital in 1974 following the death of Ken Royes. He walked off the job in 1976 when the Jamaican Ministry of Health refused to confirm him in the post. Dr. Lindsay now has a flourishing psychiatric practice in the State of Alabama in the USA. He came to see me a few years ago when he was in Jamaica on a visit. He described to me how he had left Jamaica in 1976 following the government's refusal to confirm him in the post at Bellevue. Neither of us could understand why. He was eminently qualified, he had the years of service, and his family had the right connections with the ruling political party. Trevor said that he had left Jamaica in disgust (shades of granduncle Hopetoun in 1919). Could it have been because Trevor was a dark-skinned Black man? To many this might seem almost ludicrous, but Jamaica was at that time still struggling with the legacy of self-racism which had been left us by our colonial forefathers. The time had not yet come in Jamaica when it was appropriate and acceptable for very Black people to manage large enterprises. Bear in mind that the first Black employee of a bank in Jamaica was not appointed until 1959.

Trevor described how difficult it had been for him to be able to practice in the USA after turning his back on his homeland. He had to literally go back to medical school to be able to take the exams which would qualify him to practice as a doctor in that country, and then complete a psychiatry residency training program before he could even think of setting up in practice as a psychiatrist. We remarked on the paradox of the fact that so many of Jamaica's best brains, after years of investment and study by the Jamaican people, were forced to migrate because the people in authority in all walks of life would not make room for them to live and work in their homeland. Lunatic and ludicrous as it seems, the brain drain to the North America and Europe is actually encouraged by the way in which the social system operates in Jamaica. Hidden prejudices and biases make seemingly sane administrators create enormous barriers for qualified Jamaicans either working in or wishing to return to Jamaica, to find jobs in their homeland. Certainly a product of colonialism, the present generation of leaders in Jamaica and the Caribbean do not seem to be able to tolerate the competition of younger, brighter, and better trained people being given an opportunity to share the stage with them. Nor do many seem capable of preparing successors for leadership and effectively passing power and leadership on.

Trevor Lindsay tried valiantly during his period of leadership to break the colonial stranglehold on Bellevue Hospital. He certainly played his part in helping to change mental health legislation, and he tried to transform the colonial culture of the mental hospital. We were the only two consultant psychiatrists in government service at the time. But the task was just too vast, and the resources too meagre. The more he tried to change things, the more they remained the same. At the time I had become frustrated with the lack of progress in the transformation of the hospital. There were nearly three thousand inmates in the institution at the time, with only two consultant psychiatrists and three medical officers and a handful of trained registered nurses who were expected to bring about the change.

I think that at this stage I should say something about the position of SMO at Bellevue. Under the colonial system of government, and under mental health legislation, theoretically and practically, that position was one of the most powerful in the land. Because the SMO at Bellevue had the legal power to detain anybody against their will and without recourse to law (the Mental Hospital Act of 1873 did not recognize review tribunals as a counter to unlawful detention as did the 1959 English

Mental Health Act), it was theoretically possible for the SMO to detain the Prime Minister against his will! This was so because under British Colonial Law there was no Prime Minister, only a Colonial Governor, who was the only person who had the power under law to appoint the SMO at Bellevue, the Chief of Police, and the Chief Justice. There was no post of Prime Minister in Jamaica before the Declaration of Independence in 1962. So, by law, in Jamaica, the SMO had to answer only to one person in that country, namely the Governor-General, who had replaced the Colonial Governor.

Few people in the country were aware of this conundrum. However, there was no denying the awesome power and responsibility of the role. No other SMO in the country had this power or authority, as they had to adhere to the laws governing the Ministry of Health. As statutory law, the Mental Hospital Act took precedence over the common law, which meant that the SMO was one of the most powerful persons in the state. Trevor Lindsay understood this. He had been tutored by Vincent Williams, who was even more aware of this awesome power when he occupied the post. This is one of the things which had got Trevor into trouble with the political authorities of the land.

Bellevue Hospital was situated on one hundred acres of prime land in the heart of Kingston, in the constituency of the then prime minister, Michael Manley. In the early days of his government, Manley and his Minister of Housing had simply 'captured' 20 acres of land to the east of the Bellevue property, built a number of prefabricated houses on it, almost overnight, and moved in some of the most loyal supporters of the governing party. A number of the most active, vocal, and volatile political activists thus became neighbors of the mental hospital in a Jamaica which had become incredibly tribalized and politically explosive. In a very real sense, many of them were much more 'dangerous' than the inmates of the hospital. Society was turning inside out! In 1976 Trevor Lindsay made the mistake of bringing the 'awesome power' of the SMO into a confrontational position with the new political leaders of the land, many of whom were determined to remove all vestiges of colonial power from the country. Trevor tried to get the residents of 'Dunkirk' (the name give to the new community) removed. The government, as previously mentioned, refused to confirm him in post and so he left the job, Bellevue Hospital and Jamaica in a seething rage.

I was appointed to act as Senior Medical Officer after Lindsay's departure in 1976. I was the only other qualified psychiatrist in government service at the time. There was fierce opposition to my appointment, but as I was aware of the role's recent history I informed the authorities that if I had not been confirmed in the post by the end of the year, I would revert to my substantive role in the hospital as the consultant psychiatrist responsible for rehabilitation. There was an international battle going on for the minds of the people of Jamaica at that time—some would say for the minds of African people around the world—and finding a suitably qualified psychiatrist for the institution was nigh impossible. I was appointed as SMO in December 1976. I refused to take the road taken by granduncle Hopetoun sixty years before.

I met Professor Sanford Cohen, former chair of psychiatry at the Boston University School of Medicine [9], when I gave a lecture there in 1980 organized by my classmate, psychiatrist Dr. Gerald Groves. Intrigued by the idea of 'cultural therapy', he visited Jamaica and Bellevue Hospital with his wife some months later to witness the process. Amazed at the performance and the dynamic within the community, he declared vehemently that I would never be able to write it down. This document is my attempt to prove him wrong!

Fred Hickling, Jack's Hill, Jamaica, December 2019

Bibliography

1. Hickling FW (1980) Poem "Mind Chains" from sociodrama '*Madaptations*', Bellevue Hospital (Unpublished).
2. Coates, CO (2012) Educational Developments in the British West Indies: A Historical Overview. *Semantic Scholar*, Corpus ID: 157260788.
3. Gordon S (1963) *A Century of West Indian Education*. London: Longmans, p. 15.
4. Bacchus MK (1994) *Education as and for Legitimacy: Developments in West Indian Education Between 1846 and 1895*. Ontario, Canada: Wilfrid Laurier University Press.
5. Bryan PE (2004) *The legacy of a Goldsmith—A History of Wolmer's Schools, 1729–2003*. Kingston, Jamaica: Arawak Publications.
6. Hobsbawm E (1999) *Industry and Empire: The Birth of the Industrial Revolution*, rev. ed. New York: New Press.
7. Hickling FW (2009) The European-American Psychosis: A Psychohistoriographic Perspective of Contemporary Western Civilization. *The Journal of Psychohistory. A Publication of the Institute for Psychohistory, 37*(1): 67–81.

8. Hill SA (n.d.) *Who's Who in Jamaica 1922–1924. A Biennial Bibliographic Record Containing Careers of the Principal Public Men and Women in Jamaica*. Kingston, Jamaica: The Gleaner Company Ltd.
9. Marquard B (2013) Dr. Sanford Cohen, 85; former BU Psychiatry Chairman. *Boston Globe*, October 3. https://www.bostonglobe.com/metro/2013/10/02/sanford-cohen-former-psychiatry-chairman-was-pioneer-studying-mind-body-equation-for-illness/h0EhwIhDw7ItFX1UCK7ZqM/story.html.

CHAPTER 2

The History of Madness in Jamaica 1494–1960

Why do we think Westminster's system
Left by Limey as he withdrew
Will really solve our problems
For our ship and all its crew? [1]

The history of madness has never been told for us Black people. To a large extent, it is only White people who have told the history of madness of Black people; who have written the journals of psychiatric history; who have written the textbooks of madness that define what is sanity and what is madness for us Black people. It is White folk who have classified the behavior of Black folk as being mad, who have built the asylums to contain what they define as lunacy, who have structured the laws that have dictated the configuration of the thoughts of Black folk. Relentlessly, the Whites continue to define our madness. It was the prominent White American physician Dr. Samuel Cartwright in 1851 who described 'Drapetomania' as a mental illness causing unruly Black slaves to run away from captivity [2]. It was Cartwright (1793–1863), born in Fairfax County, Virginia, a physician who practiced in Mississippi and Louisiana, who scripted *Dysaesthesia Aethiopica* as 'hebetude of the mind and obtuse sensibility of the body—a disease peculiar to Negroes—called by overseers, "rascality"'. It was Cartwright who opined that this disease is 'the natural offspring of Negro liberty—the liberty to be idle, to wallow in filth, and to indulge in improper food and drinks'.

F. W. Hickling, *Decolonization of Psychiatry in Jamaica*,
https://doi.org/10.1007/978-3-030-48489-7_2

We Black folk continue to allow White people to be the creators of our insanity; to define us as schizophrenic; and to shape our psychopathy. Systematically, relentlessly, flying in the face of all reason, we have allowed these White people to capture us, to transport us, to enslave us, to exploit us, and to keep us enchained in their ghettos, in their prisons, and in their lunatic asylums. It was Benjamin Rush (1746–1813), 'The Father of American Psychiatry,' whose portrait was on the official seal of the American Psychiatric Association until 2015, signer of the Declaration of Independence of the USA, Dean of the Medical School at the University of Pennsylvania, who described Black people as suffering from a genetic affliction called *Negritude*, akin to the disease of leprosy [3]. Samuel Cartwright was an apprentice of Benjamin Rush. From those days until the present, White physicians have been defining the madness of Black people and inventing cruel and inhumane treatments to treat our so-called lunacy.

Europeans have written most accounts of the history of madness in Jamaica and the Caribbean. There is little documentation about mental illness in Black people before the beginning of the nineteenth century. Most written histories of madness begin the discourse with the Greeks and identify the Greek physician Hippocrates (460–377 BC) as being the first recorded author of madness becoming the object of scientific speculation. The discourse usually identifies Aristotle, Galen, and Plato as architects of the idea of madness in the European dominant medical model. The historical treatise usually meanders through the Roman Empire, the Middle Ages, and the European Renaissance through the age of Enlightenment into the modern era, lionizing Philippe Pinel (1745–1826) and Jean-Étienne Dominique Esquirol (1772–1840) in France, Wiiliam Tuke (1732–1822) and Samuel Tuke (1784–1857) in England, and Emil Kraepelin (1856–1926), Karl Jaspers (1883–1969), and Sigmund Freud (1856–1939) in Germany and Austria as the forerunners of contemporary psychiatry. In the contemporary literature on the history of madness or of psychiatry in the world, it appears as if the world consists of nowhere but Europe. Based on the documentation of mental illness and its treatment, the continents of Africa, India, South America, and China do not seem to exist.

The early sixteenth-century writings of the Spanish friar, Bartolomé de las Casas, made the earliest reference to madness of the indigenous people in the New World in 1542 as he described the encounter with the practices of the indigenous Taino in Jamaica and the Caribbean. He noted that a form of community psychiatry was practiced by the Taino before European colonization of the region. Las Casas describes how the mentally ill of that period were allowed to wander at large and were fed by the local population, and treated with unguents and salves and herbal potions. But perhaps more poignantly, he identified the madness of the European colonizers of the New World with profound clarity, describing the genocidal madness of the Spanish invaders as the most profound expression of psychopathology of the White nations of the world [4], perpetrating egregious robberies and villainies including unheard of cruelties by murdering, burning, roasting, and exposing men to be torn to pieces by dogs.

The European encounter with the New World began as an accident with Christopher Columbus endeavoring to find a passage to the Far East. Instead of finding it, he encountered millions and millions of human beings, unknown to the European world, who inhabited North and South America and the Caribbean. Jamaica was 'discovered' by Columbus in 1494 and was initially colonized by Spain, whose interests were focused almost entirely on the discovery and exploitation of the mineral resources of silver and gold. What the Spanish found instead was a contented, peace-loving, pliable Taino population with a self-reliant society, and an absence of precious metals. The work of Charles Duff [5], who translated the diaries of Columbus's three voyages to the New World, makes no equivocation about the symptoms of delusions and madness that exemplified Columbus's writings and behavior. He wrote that Columbus had a megalomaniac's craving for power and his extraordinary imagination produced hallucinations, visions, and day-dreams, and that he mentioned at least two occasions on which 'voices' spoke to him. Duff wrote that from the moment Columbus had become obsessed by his great idea of discovering the 'Land to the West,' there was no feat of lying, exaggeration, misrepresentation, and hypocrisy to which he did not rise to achieve his goal. He suggested that Columbus was capable of sharp practice and utmost dishonesty, callousness, and even of cruelty. It was Columbus, Duff (ibid., pp. 263–265) suggested, who initiated the dreadful gold levy on the Indians and thereby became responsible for a bad example which was followed by long years of cruelty afterward.

The antithetical perception of this 'discovery' by the Europeans is strongly contested by the perceptions of the indigenous Caribbean and American people, who regarded the European 'discovery' much more as an intrusion and in reality as an invasion of their personal, social, and geographic space by marauding White pirates. Las Casas identifies the antithetical processes involved in this period and the murderous psychopathology of the Spaniards: '...on a sudden, some wicked Devil possessing the minds of the Spaniards, agitated them with great fury...' The Europeans were singularly interested in plunder and the exploitation of the human, mineral, and other treasures of the lands that they had found. The principal insight of Columbus's offensive intrusion was the realization of the Eurocentric concept of *White supremacy*, which asserted European ownership of the world and the people and resources therein by divine right. These were the elements of a collective insanity which I have called the *European psychosis* [6, 7]. Essential to this perception was that people of color, indigenous inhabitants of the rest of the world, were sub-human, only slightly superior to domestic animals. The Three-Fifths Compromise was an accommodation reached in the fledgling USA between delegates from the Southern states and Northern states during the 1787 American Constitutional Convention. Delegates (and Founding Fathers) James Wilson (1742–1798) and Roger Sherman (1721–1793)[1, 2] proposed the arrangement. The Three-Fifths Compromise is found in Article 1, Section 2, Paragraph 3 of the United States Constitution which reads:

> ...Representatives and direct Taxes shall be apportioned among the several States which may be included within this Union, according to their respective Numbers, which shall be determined by adding to the whole Number of free Persons, including those bound to service for a term of years, and excluding Indians not taxed, *three fifths of all other Persons*... [8]

A contentious issue at the Constitutional Convention was whether slaves would be counted as part of the population in determining representation of the States in the Congress or would instead be considered property and, as such, not be considered for purposes of representation. The debate was over if, and if so, how, slaves would be counted when determining a state's total population for legislative representation and taxing purposes. The issue was important, as this population number would then be used to determine the number of seats that the state would have in the United States House of Representatives for the next ten years, and to determine what percentage of the nation's direct tax burden each state would have to bear [8].

This was the essence of the European madness with which they populated the New World. Clearly, these ideas of owning the land and the people of the world were out of keeping with the belief systems of almost every culture in the world with the exception of the aristocratic ruling class European culture. Kevin Cahill has reported that the world's primary feudal landowner is Queen Elizabeth II. She is Queen of 32 countries, head of a Commonwealth of 54 countries in which a quarter of the world's population lives, and legal owner of about 6.6 billion acres of land, one-sixth of the earth's land surface [9].

By means of the systematic eradication of all opposition of the indigenous people by mindless and ferocious genocide, the Europeans were able to impose the madness of European colonization on the world. Las Casas described the ruthless and cruel genocidal destruction of the gentle inhabitants of Jamaica by the Spanish colonizers, who had wiped out the entire population of two million, with only seventy-four remaining by 1611 [10]. Millions of people were wiped out not only by disease brought to the New World by the Spaniards, but also by a systematic genocidal destruction of these people who were hunted down by bounty hunters paid for by the state. The Spanish were excited by the prospect of gold and other mineral riches to be found in the New World. By the middle of the seventeenth century, the Caribbean island of Jamaica, which had been inhabited by more than a million Arawak Indians when Columbus invaded one hundred and fifty years before, had been reduced in its population to ten thousand people, eight thousand of whom were Spaniards. The indigenous Taino and Kalinago (Caribs) island people of the Caribbean (related to the Kalina Mainland Caribs of South America) were ruthlessly and systematically eradicated genocidally by the Spanish colonizers of the sixteenth century. Only tiny populations of Carib Indians presently remain in the islands of Dominica and Tobago [11] in the eastern Caribbean. Genocide is a murderous madness that promises complete and total political domination of a social space by the lunatics that carry out such massacres. Genocide means not just mass killing, to the level of extermination, but mass obliteration to the verge of extinction [12].

Following the extermination of the indigenous Caribbean and New World people, the European countries of Britain, Spain, France, and Holland quickly divided the Americas and the Caribbean territories among themselves and instituted the next expression of European madness in the New World—the systematic implementation of African slavery via the Middle Passage, bringing millions of Black Africans to fuel the plantation economy, which spawned the capitalist economic system [13] that they had created. The European psychosis had been dragged into reality by the genocidal negation of the cultural opposition. The gun had become the midwife of the madness.

The British captured Jamaica in 1655 with a force led by William Penn and Robert Venables after an unsuccessful attempt to seize Santo Domingo from the Spanish as part of Oliver Cromwell's 'grand design.' The vast majority of the people who initially shaped this country, the rest of the West Indies, and the New World came against their will. This was true not only of the African slaves, but also of the large numbers of Irish, Welsh, Scottish, and English migrants, who came initially as indentured servants and later as a result of the pressures of economic exploitation in Britain. General Venables described the English soldiers he commanded as a rascally rabble of raw and inexperienced men, apprentices who had fled their masters or who had spent time in jail. It is unlikely that this motley rabble, initially at least, were willing participants in the European psychosis; however, they may well have come to appreciate the benefits to be reaped from adhering to such delusionary beliefs and practices and experienced a conversion.

It is truly amazing that the European genocide of the New World and the monumental enslavement of millions of Africans by Europeans in the fifteenth to the nineteenth centuries never enter into the discourse about the history of madness written predominantly by European scholars. The untold physical and mental suffering of the enslaved African people in that period must have been horrendous. But whoever heard of a mad slave? Slaves who had physical and mental disabilities would no doubt have been swiftly executed and exterminated by their murderous European slave owners and slave masters, leaving the perception that mental illness was something that was not known in African people. There is no mention of the imposition of slavery as a cause of insanity in any historical discourse of madness that has originated in the European world. It is as if that event and period of history have simply vanished, or have had no psychological or psychiatric effect on the slaver or the slave. It is *as if* the theft of millions of Black men, women, and children from their homes in Africa, and the subjugation of these stolen people, forced to endure a ten- to twelve-week punishing and brutal voyage across the Atlantic with starvation rations in inhuman travelling conditions, was really a trifling inconvenience leaving few physical or psychological sequelae on the perpetrators or the victims. This has left a profound blindness in the thinking, reasoning, or writings of contemporary Europeans. To the European malefactors, and the Europeans who have subsequently chronicled the history of madness, four-fifths of the world's population and culture seemed not to exist. The question has to be asked: how has the European world of the past five hundred years seen the existence of madness in the non-European peoples? Did the Europeans in this period recognize the coping mechanisms and therapeutic management skills exhibited by these populations in addressing the mental pathology that must have arisen during the periods of slavery and colonialism? Is Europe conscious of the egregious effects of their deliberate social engineering practices on the Africans that they enslaved in the New World? In a disturbing, brilliant account of the consequences of European imperialism in Africa, Swedish historian Sven Lindqvist manages to document the genocidal intent of the European colonizer from the sixteenth century as a calculated and deliberate attempt to obliterate people of color, in order to establish White European domination of the world. Lindqvist opined that, in practice, the whole of Europe acted according to the maxim 'Exterminate all the brutes.' Officially, it was of course denied: 'But man to man, everyone knew…no one doubted it' [14].

The birth of modern racism began with the invasion of the New World by King Ferdinand V and Queen Isabella, the architects of the Spanish Inquisition, with the Catholic Church as the wet nurse [15]. Genocidal eradication of the inhabitants of the New World and the institution of African slavery by marauding Europeans established the foundations of present-day Western civilization. Charles Duff in *The Truth About Columbus* estimated that in this terrible episode of human history about twelve million Amerindians disappeared forever from the face of the earth [5]. The extermination of the indigenous population of the Caribbean set the stage for the arrival of slaves from Africa. Carew suggested that by the time the slaves from Africa began arriving in the Americas, the European colonizers' appetite for untrammelled cruelty, individual and collective sadism, and an unbridled greed for gold had already been titillated by the extermination of millions of native Americans [15].

The political history of the New World is replete with instances of the measured social engineering of European colonizers designed to influence popular attitudes and social behaviors on a large scale. Imperial European governments, media, politicians, and private groups have wantonly used Machiavellian social engineering techniques to design and methodically influence social events to facilitate their intent. Once the social event triggered a successful outcome, it was repeated again and again with the aim of escalating the desired outcome. One of the earliest records of the psychological social engineering methods employed by the British colonizers came from Willie Lynch, who was a British slave owner from Barbados. He was invited to the colony of Virginia in America to teach his methods of controlling Black slaves by setting them against one another. The term 'lynching' is derived from his name. He advocated the use of *fear, distrust, and envy* for control purposes and counseled that distrust is stronger than trust; and envy is stronger than adulation, respect, or admiration. The self-refueling and self-generating indoctrination effect on the Black slave he predicted would perpetuate subjugation for hundreds of years. The document *The Making of a Slave* [16] in which these psychological control maneuvers were recommended is purportedly the record of a speech delivered to an audience on the banks of the James River in Virginia in 1712, but its historical accuracy has been challenged by White [17] and Black [18] historians in America. However, there is a saying in Jamaican dialect culture '…if it *never* go so, it *nearly* go so…,' meaning that if the described events did not entirely occur as stated, then they occurred only to a slightly lesser extent in reality!

The postcolonial psychological analytic technique of psychohistoriography was developed by the present author in 1978 to address the condition of descendants of Africans enslaved in the New World. It was designed to help people from various socioeconomic and educational backgrounds deal with underdeveloped political and psychological constructs, to debunk the myths of colonization, and to establish reality as a framework for future action. Essential to the delusion of this European psychosis was that people of color, indigenous inhabitants of the rest of the world, were sub-human, only slightly superior to domestic animals. The European psychosis has created distorted historical, political, and social images of the colonized people. The colonized have no history, their values are uncivilized, and their history of struggle against the process has not been recorded. Integral to the collective European colonial psychosis is the attempt to negate the values, culture, and social history of the colonized. A slave was simply that—a slave. He was not a farmer, a carpenter, a writer, or a healer. She was not an artist, a jeweler, a historian, or a nurse. He/she was depersonalized—he/she was a slave. He/she had no name and took the name of the slave owner. Within the ideology of this European psychosis, the colonizer set up political, legal, social, and economic institutions that facilitated the process of continuous individual and collective underdevelopment. There exists a gigantic scotoma or blind spot in the psychic understanding of Europeans to the physical and psychological trauma that was perpetrated by their wanton wholesale theft and imperialistic enslavement of Africa and the New World, and virtually a total miscomprehension of their etiologic role in world economics and psychopathology played by their wanton genocide of people of color. Their initial response was to ignore or deny the existence of the mental illness perpetrated by their callous ruthlessness. During the period of slavery in the Caribbean, which extended from the early sixteenth to the mid-nineteenth century, the health of slaves was the responsibility of the slave owners. Mentally ill slaves, as recorded by Las Casas, were housed in plantation dungeons called 'hothouses' in deplorable and horrendous conditions. Between the late seventeenth century and emancipation, a violently mentally ill slave would invariably be executed rather than rehabilitated. Torture of slaves in the West Indies may have surpassed the concomitant draconian treatment of the mentally ill in European asylums. The slave master had absolute power over the slave, with many documented cases of slave masters barbarously butchering their slaves without redress or punishment [19].

The arrogant racist perception of many European doctors at the time was that mental illness was rare in Black people due to poor mental development. In a report to the British Parliament, the learned physician Sir Andrew Halliday [20] wrote that he seldom met with insanity among the savage tribes of men, with not one of his African travelers remarking their having seen a single madman. He opined that among the slaves in the West Indies madness very rarely occurs. However, the reality is that there was a high incidence of mental illness in the Africans enslaved in the New World, and suicide [21] in defiance to the collective trauma of slavery was prevalent. Hickling [22] quoting from Orlando Patterson [23], in a historical review of psychiatry in the Anglophone Caribbean, reported that mass suicides of groups of 25 or more African slaves were regular occurrences, and cases of outright insanity caused by the impact of the conditions on board the slave ships had been reported. Facilities for treating such mental illness were virtually non-existent in that period. The rudimentary hospitals or 'hothouses' on some slave plantations were used for solitary confinement. The high numbers of 'weakly' or invalid slaves were an indication of the cruel treatment and extremely severe labor to which the Africans were subjected [22].

Suicide by hanging and dirt eating [22] at an individual and a group level was a common reaction to slavery among Black Africans within the Caribbean plantation system. William Fitzmaurice, a planter resident in Jamaica between 1771 and 1788, reported: 'I lost in one year a dozen new Negroes by dirt eating, though I fed them well—when I remonstrated with them, they constantly told me that they preferred dying to living; and a great proportion of the new Negroes who go upon sugar plantations die in this manner' [23]. Lester [21] reported the story of a slave named Dominico who was required to work in the sugar mill even though his illnesses made it impossible. He tried to persuade the overseer that he could not work, whereupon he was given twenty-five lashes. The same punishment was administered in the next two days. Dominico then went to the mill and asked the workers to stir up the fires, after which he threw himself into the machines and was crushed to death (quoted from Blassingame, p. 257 [24]). Since almost all slaves were brutally treated, punishment per se seems insufficient as a cause of suicide, but slavery itself seems to be an a priori cause of suicide in African slaves.

But the horrors of the African experience in the New World did nothing to diminish the African cunning for survival, wisdom for regeneration and reinvention of self, penchant for adaptation, and courage to resist the racist crime against humanity that was African enslavement. Africans showed a stubborn refusal to accept the status of slaves. It seems clear that from the inception of slavery in the Caribbean the Black slaves could not rely on the efficacy of the facilities provided by the slave master or the colonial government for their health treatment and care. Clearly, the colonial masters were out of touch with the mental health needs of the Africans who were enslaved in the New World and were unwilling or unable to recognize their psychological condition. Mental health facilities provided by the British at that time simply continued the tradition of violence and restraint which had started with the Spanish colonialists. Mid-eighteenth century records of the slave court of the parish of St. Andrew, Jamaica, enable scholars to analyze the crimes for which slaves were prosecuted and the judicial punishments they received [25]. Prosecutions concentrated heavily on a few offenses, especially theft and running away. Punishments were severe and were largely concerned with the slave's body; they included death, flogging, transportation, and bod ily mutilation. Some punishments made use of the cotton tree *(Ceiba pentandra)*, which figured significantly in Afro-Jamaican cosmology, suggesting that the authorities were trying to harness or combat the power of Obeah [25]. Certainly, any form of violent behavior (psychiatric or otherwise) was treated with the legal penalty of death [25] often in a barbarous manner, such as slow burning. In 1760 after Tacky's Rebellion, some insurgents were burned alive and others gibbetted alive, left to die in prolonged agony [26].

Traditional healing practices were the norm for the slave population of the Caribbean, who also had to rely on their traditional healers for the care of their mental illnesses. Traditional religious beliefs (and medicine) in the Caribbean have taken many names such as Kumina and Myalism in Jamaica, Shango and Orisha in Trinidad, Cumfeh in Guyana, Santeria in Cuba, Vodou in Haiti, and Obeah all over the region [27]. The colonial powers were genuinely intimidated by the power of Obeah and other African belief systems, the British using every means at their disposal to control it and stamp it out. The plantation owners forbade the practice of Obeah, banning the drum and other cultural forms of expression. It was outlawed in Jamaica in 1760 and it remains illegal today. In later years, committed believers and practitioners were often incarcerated in the lunatic asylum.

The enslaved African people in the New World have always resisted slavery, using every means at their command, and in spite of the repressive nature of British colonialism. Jamaica stands out as the colony with the highest numbers of slave rebellions. The slaves in Jamaica were never docile and accepting of their lot—they were warlike and resorted to any means to obtain a better way of life. No matter what forces conspired against them, the Blacks never ceased in their struggle to be treated as human beings. They struggled for human dignity, recognizing that the White colonizer was destroying their African culture. Elements of their culture had disappeared in the oceans of the Middle Passage. But the memory of Africa was powerful and energized their collective struggle. They had come from a great civilization that had endured for millennia. African people had their own kings and queens, their own religions and universities, and their own culinary traditions and artistic heritage. The first struggle of Africans enslaved in the New World was how to preserve and enrich their culture in the face of the domination of the European psychosis that was justified by most of the leading European academics and intellectuals. The struggle of Black people through slavery and beyond has always been for the basic necessities of food, clothing, and shelter, which would then be buttressed by demands for freedom, land ownership, employment, better wages and working conditions, health, and education—the necessary requirements for human survival and development. But this pattern of revolutionary violence to overcome the European psychosis did not stop with emancipation; it has continued unabated till the present time, precisely because the European psychosis is alive and well today and still continues to oppress, vilify, and denigrate Black people around the world. A cyclical pattern of violent rebellion in Jamaica can be traced through the historical record of the Spanish Negro Slave revolt of 1663, the First Maroon War led by Cudjoe in 1728–40, the Nanny Rebellion of 1730, Tacky's Rebellion in 1760, the Second Maroon War of 1795–96, and the Sam Sharpe Rebellion of 1831–32 [28]. Starting in the 1660s as a struggle of Black people against the crushing madness of the European psychosis, it has continued up to the gas riots (triggered by rises in the price of gasoline) in 1985 and 1999 [29].

Recent European accounts of madness in Jamaica and the Caribbean usually ignore the overwhelming evidence of monstrous behavior displayed by the colonizers and the horrendous and complex trauma experienced by the Africans enslaved in the New World. Complex trauma has been identified and accepted as a potent causative factor in contemporary psychiatry [30] and has been normalized in contemporary Caribbean culture as being interchangeable with the maintenance of discipline and order. Flogging was regarded as a simple form of punishment threat the childlike Blacks could understand and was seen as a justifiably powerful deterrent that was the mainstay punishment in the colonial constitution for minor crimes [24]. European historians usually begin the discourse on the history of madness with the construction of the Lunatic Asylum in 1861. This is utterly disingenuous at best and unequivocally dishonest at worst. With the African slave emancipation struggle gaining ground in Europe and America by the beginning of the nineteenth century, the slave owners in the colonies were forced to take into consideration the health of their slaves and the provision of health care for them.

The Post-Emancipation Period: Circa 1834–1900

Jamaica's first lunatic asylum was established in 1819, comprising 12 single cells next to the Public Hospital in Kingston. The facility provided primarily for White Jamaicans. By 1840, that asylum contained over 80 inmates, its racial composition having altered significantly in the wake of emancipation. A committee of the House of Assembly highlighted its grossly overcrowded and insanitary conditions. The disgraceful state of both institutions was brought firmly into the public domain in 1858 by the efforts of Jamaican-born Dr. Lewis Quier Bowerbank, a prominent White Kingston physician. Twenty years previously, £10,000 had been voted to construct a new asylum, and an experienced English asylum architect, John Conolly [31] was commissioned to design a building for 250 people. However, due to a toxic combination of unregulated expenditure, corruption, political ineptitude, and design flaws, it did not actually open for another twenty years.

Bowerbank mounted a fierce campaign against the hospital's authorities, medical officers, and subordinate staff, exposing the various evils and abuses that prevailed. His campaign brought extensive newspaper coverage, the publication of trenchant pamphlets on behalf of various protagonists, and even prosecutions of staff for neglect and cruelty [32, 33]. The conditions for the mentally ill incarcerated in the asylum in Kingston were appalling. The situation of overcrowding and ill treatment that existed in that institution was recorded by the Warden of the time as constituting 'a chamber of horrors' [34], and the physical abuses commonly inflicted on the patients of that institution were described by Henry Taylor, the Head of the West Indian Department at the Colonial Office, as 'most cruel and revolting crimes' [35]. Bowerbank took his crusade all the way to London, successfully enlisting the support of Lord Shaftesbury and the Commissioners in Lunacy. The scandal of the Jamaica Lunatic Asylum received widespread attention in medical journals like *The Lancet* [36] and in the most influential newspaper, *The Times* [37]. British liberal public opinion was outraged by this apparent disgrace to the ideals of Empire, in a colony expected to set an enlightened example of the recovery from slavery after abolition.

In Jamaica, in 1861, impetus was given to the opening of the long-delayed new asylum at Rae's Town, on the seafront outside Kingston. The male patients were transferred from the old asylum in November 1860, and the females eventually followed in the autumn of 1862. A statue was built to honor Bowerbank and was initially located in a prominent position on the Kingston waterfront at the foot of King Street, the main boulevard of the colonial city. At the height of the worker rebellion against British colonial rule in 1938, irate Jamaican workers showed the contempt that they felt for Bowerbank by stoning the statue, thereby removing the nose and part of the face. The statue was moved for safety to the grounds of Bellevue Hospital, where it remains today.

The development of lunatic asylums around the world in the eighteenth and nineteenth centuries heralded the European colonial creation of custodial institutions to contain the violence unleashed by this period of colonial exploitation worldwide. The gross inadequacies of British imperial management revealed by the post-emancipation governance scandal concerning the treatment of patients in the asylum in Kingston in the nineteenth century were highlighted in an appraisal of the imperfect models of British postcolonial mental health policy. In an entire culture created by colonization, both the ideology of mental health and the processes for the treatment of mental illness have demanded a decolonization epistemology. The imposition of a master/slave culture for the maximization of economic exploitation of the society became the tapestry within which the recognition of conformity and subservience was woven. Counter-culturally, the inherent cultural ideology of the colonized formed the bulwark upon which the resistance and rebellion of the enslaved people emerged, challenging the very tenets of the religious, social, and emotional constructions of the colonizer. It is suggested that the development of psychiatry in the Caribbean reflects the convergence and syncretism resulting from the opposing vectors of the colonizer-colonized engagement.

One of the most prolific contemporary British writers of the history of madness in the British colonies, Leonard Smith of the University of Birmingham, has posited the need to re-evaluate British colonial history in this period, suggesting that measures to remove, sequestrate, and care for the insane were central elements in Britain's 'civilizing mission' [38]. In his recent book, Smith [39] strengthens his ameliorative position on the 'civilizing mission' and reinforces his attempt to diminish Britain's profound causative role in the social dislocation and dysfunction in the colonial territories of which he writes. He has also suggested that the English asylum system had attained a degree of sophistication in its transmission to the West Indian colonies, and that the British approach had to be adapted to meet the unique social, political, and economic circumstances of a region dominated by the complex realities and consequences associated with the enslavement of Black African people and their emancipation in 1838. Social dislocation and dysfunction were endemic all over the region and persisted, to varying degrees, throughout the period under consideration.

Smith's comments raise profound disquiet as they suggest that the birth of the asylum in the Caribbean represented a genuine British therapeutic, albeit paternalistic, response to insanity. In his review of missionary work in the West Indies published in 1828, Hope Waddell reported that the slave trade had been prosecuted by colonialists in Jamaica with the 'utmost recklessness' [40]. The asylum that Britain built in 1861 in Jamaica and the prison only half a mile away were institutions of social containment for the descendants of Africans who had been enslaved in the New World. This was the very same British government that had sought to neutralize the philosophical, psychological, and spiritual rebellion of a people brutally enslaved by imperialistic greed and colonial psychopathy and was providing anything but 'containment, care and treatment...in the English lunatic asylum system [that] had attained a degree of sophistication,' as Smith has suggested [39, p. 6]. The proliferation of asylums and workhouses reflected the harsh and draconian social conditions characteristic of this period of Britain's history and imposed by a ruling class that was driven by greed, oppression, and an appetite for social domination. Michel Foucault [41] famously construed the period in Europe beginning in the mid-seventeenth century and lasting through most of the eighteenth as the 'Great Confinement'. People who were seen as being social misfits, incapable of contributing to the labor market and earning a living, were deemed to be insane and incarcerated by the million in an organized network of custodial institutions without any recourse. Kenneth Lakritz [42] comments: 'With his Francocentric perspective, Foucault fastens particularly on an edict of 1656 that established the Hôpital général of Paris....[he] suggests that it was really a moral panic provoked by rural displacement, industrialization, and a new class of urban surplus labor'. Foucault's biting criticism of the nature of British and European society during this period has drawn into the question the real origin of insanity in Britain and Europe at that time, and disingenuous European methods of attempting to treat madness by forcible custodialization and draconian physical therapies. The reforming works of Quaker Samuel Tuke (founder of 'moral treatment' at the York Retreat in England) and Philippe Pinel (representative of the French Revolution, who reorganized the French hospitals—symbolically breaking the chains shackling the inmates of the Salpêtrière) were attacked by Foucault as 'a gigantic moral imprisonment' [42]. Lakritz suggests, however, that perhaps Foucault's greatest influence has produced the Western contemporary 'Great Deconfinement'—the emptying of the state psychiatric hospitals with the achievement that the mentally ill are once again 'free to beg in the streets and sleep under bridges'—paraphrasing the now famous quote of another French author, Anatole France: 'The law, in its majestic equality, forbids rich as well as the poor to sleep under bridges, beg in the streets, and to steal bread' [43].

The trenchant analysis by Margaret Jones of the appalling conditions endured by patients at the asylum in Kingston cogently explodes Smith's ameliorative claims of Britain's mental health 'civilizing mission.' She described that most notorious of the 'most cruel and revolting crimes' was the practice of tanking—forcibly holding patients under water. Following the death of a patient in the asylum, the matron and two nurses were charged with manslaughter. Although they were acquitted by the jury, the case erupted into a public scandal. Jones explored the insights that this shameful episode offers on Jamaica's colonial past, by exposing the fractures between the Jamaican governing classes and the imperial government and revealing the internal divisions within colonial society. The low level of government commitment to the health of the Jamaican people was reflected in the poor conditions at the asylum and was a legacy of slavery [35].

Smith has also written extensively about the concept of 'moral treatment' and the role of British physician Dr. Thomas Allen in introducing the concept in the Jamaica Lunatic Asylum [39]. The Jamaican understanding of the history of Allen exposes this disingenuousness. Allen was appointed to the asylum in 1863. Undoubtedly, as Smith and others have described, he introduced the principles of 'moral treatment' and 'non-restraint' pioneered by Tuke. Allen had previously instituted them as part of an extensive program of patient employment at the Lincolnshire County Lunatic Asylum while working there as Assistant Medical Officer.

But there was a darker side to Allen's therapeutic practices, which reflected the contempt in which he held Black Jamaican people. This institutionalized racism was shared by many of the colonial doctors who followed him. Allen had a particularly cruel and vindictive racist streak that was disguised behind the prevailing colonial ethos of the 'civilizing process' of the Black Jamaican people. We must remember that the lunatic asylum of the 1860s provided treatment for the White ruling class and Brown middle class, who were treated in quite a different fashion from the Black agricultural workers. Most people at home in Jamaica and abroad are unaware that there were extensive and separate private wards in the old Male and Female Divisions of Bellevue Hospital, which disappeared following postcolonial deinstitutionalization in the 1970s. I can bear witness to these facilities that were dismantled soon after I joined the hospital's staff. This apartheid construct, inherited from the Jamaica Lunatic Asylum that I found when I started working at Bellevue, was likely to have been imposed by Allen, who had attracted money later in his tenure to expedite the building of additional rooms and wards at the asylum to initiate his proposal to Governor Grant and the Colonial Office to separate the more dangerous patients from the 'harmless cases' [44]. None of the descriptions that I have read of the asylum around this time mentions this 'apartheid architecture'. Smith [39, p. 87] describes in detail the building of separate wards with single rooms on the male and female sides of the asylum. This was certainly reflected in the architectural divisions that I encountered when I arrived in the early 1970s. However, there was no mention of the wards reserved exclusively for the White- and Brown-skinned admissions.

Thomas Allen had, it seems, brought about a remarkable transformation in the institution within a relatively short time. However, he had created a paternalistic, colonial, apartheid-like mini-society within the asylum's walls. He had a clear vision of what he wanted to achieve, and what the obstacles were. His autocratic, paternalistic, and obsessional nature has been reported by the various chroniclers mentioned here. The asylum that I witnessed as a young medical officer mirrored perfectly the apartheid-like structure of Jamaican society.

He was not averse to taking a stand even if it meant falling out with the Colonial Governor. An early supporter was Governor Edward John Eyre, who departed Jamaica after the 1865 Morant Bay debacle [45]. This was the seventh in the thirty-year cycle of violent Jamaican rebellions starting in 1663 [28]. The Morant Bay Rebellion, led by George William Gordon and Paul Bogle, came hard on the heels of the Great Baptist Revival. Paul Bogle, himself a Baptist deacon, marched with his followers in response to grievances over land and the maladministration of justice. Characteristically, the reaction of the colonial administration was brutal and swift. Eyre, who had been sent to Australia in the 1840s, had shown paternalistic solicitude toward the Aborigines, whom he constructed as 'poor untutored children of impulse... misjudged and misrepresented by English settlers who were maltreating them and deserving of care and the improvements of civilization from whites.' Having Lake Eyre in South Australia named after him was his reward. However, after his success in Australia, he was appointed Governor of

Jamaica and supervised a murderous 30-day rampage by his troops, killing 439 people, flogging 600 others, and burning over 1000 homes of suspected rebels. This after he mistook a local riot for a full-scale uprising. What had changed from the benevolent paternalism he had exhibited in Australia? He now encountered Black people who demanded membership in the world and were prepared to demonstrate their right to property and respect. Governor Eyre now described West Indian Blacks as savages without culture, who needed to be mastered by White men [46].

The Colonial Governor's brutal reaction to the Morant Bay Rebellion resounded in Whitehall. A controversy developed between those who felt that Eyre's reaction was in keeping with the nature of British colonialism and its insistence on law and order, and those who felt that his conduct was nothing short of the brutality of a tyrant. Eyre was removed from the governorship after being tried in court. Sir John Peter Grant succeeded him, and Jamaica was converted to Crown colony government. Grant quickly reacted to the situation by driving squatters from the land and then setting up the (semi-military) Jamaica Constabulary Force and Rural Police Force. A public system of elementary education was also started, roads and bridges were built, and a public medical service was established. In spite of these ameliorative gestures, the economic and social conditions continued to deteriorate. In early 1869, Allen found himself in dispute with Grant. Later in the year, there were strong rumors circulating that Allen had been suspended by Grant, due to 'serious differences' between them, though this could not be substantiated.

Despite his progressive reforms and paternalistic approach, Allen's perspective had remained unaltered. Indeed, his position had probably hardened, along with the attitudes of the White ruling elite, in the wake of Morant Bay [47]. In 1874, he suggested that the 'brutal condition of an uncivilised community makes it a matter of accident whether the individual be consigned to a Lunatic Asylum or a Prison.' In either case, it was 'their ungovernable passions and brutal tendencies' that prevented their being allowed to 'remain at large with safety to the community' [48].

Thomas Allen's successful work in Jamaica was becoming widely known and in 1874 it was proposed that he be appointed Inspector for Lunatic Asylums in the West Indies [39: 88, 229]. The Barbados inspection did not produce the outcome that Allen had anticipated. His painstaking approach to the task brought lengthy delays in producing a report, which did not finally appear for more than a year. In 1876 the report on the Barbados Asylum finally appeared [49]; it was highly critical, exposing major deficiencies in every conceivable aspect of its operation. It also gave him the opportunity to expound his ideas regarding race. He repeated the argument that the very nature of the 'negro peasantry' made many of them brutal and pathological; he attributed this to their low standard of intellect, concluding that it must be responsible for their being little more than mere 'thinking automata'. He suggested that the 'ungovernable feelings, passions, and emotions' of Negro people may render 'many fit subjects for a lunatic asylum, when there is little or no decided intellectual aberration'. The want of education and civilizing influences, he suggested, 'fails to secure the least power of self-control and may fairly be admitted as an extenuating circumstance when criminal acts are complained of'. For this reason, he suggested that there were many who should be subjected to the reforming influence of a well-regulated lunatic asylum rather than be branded as criminals [49].

Allen went on to delineate the 'vast difference between the peasantry of England, and the uncivilized negro of the West Indies,' suggesting that the 'ferocity and ungovernable passion of the Jamaican Negro is well known, and a trifling exciting cause, makes him lose all power of self control'. Allen portrayed the underlying dynamics of poor Black people in Jamaica living in the mountains 'leading a wild and savage life', far removed from any civilizing influences or European associations. This British 'moral architect' of 'moral treatment' based on occupation, organized leisure pursuits, religious participation, and personal interactions between medical men and patients, deemed that the negro was not only uneducated, but 'has wanted that experience, example, and discipline during childhood, which should fit him for the duties of society when he reached manhood. We have therefore present deplorable ignorance and superstition and besides the antagonism of race, that selfishness in all its brutality, with all its unsociability which has long been characteristic of an uncivilized people' (p. 59) [49]. Allen sought to protect insane members of the (White) middle classes from such people. He advocated separate accommodation to ensure that 'governesses, daughters of clergymen, decayed gentlewomen, and men who have been engaged in various pursuits' no longer had to mix with 'negroes or others of such savage habits,' whereby admission to the asylum became 'more a misfortune than a blessing' (p. 61) [49].

Allen turned up in London in September 1876 to press his claims to be appointed as Inspector, but several key colonies declined to participate. There were concerns about the financial costs and a resentment of outside interference, a reflection of Allen's obsessive and overbearing approach. On his return to Jamaica, he increasingly came into conflict with local officials and politicians, often about petty matters [50]. Allen acknowledged that some of the problems that arose among the patients and staff of the asylum could be attributed to the legacy of slavery within Jamaican society, citing factors like the widespread lack of formal marriage, the high incidence of 'illegitimate' births, and low levels of literacy. In consequence, there were 'immense difficulties' in maintaining 'proper efficiency and discipline,' particularly because of the untrained, undisciplined nature of the staff who were recruited [51] and who had also, by this time, managed to arouse the hostility of the local press, particularly the *Jamaica Gleaner* [52].

At the end of August 1886, nearing the end of his stay in Jamaica, he gave the Governor notice of his intention to retire. In September, despite rumors of his impending retirement, the *Gleaner* published in full a colorful letter contending that the asylum was an 'autocracy,' where the medical superintendent held 'unlimited sway' over four hundred of 'our poor, afflicted fellow citizens.' Among other charges, the writer claimed that recovered patients were kept in far longer than was necessary, so that they could continue to be employed at their trades without payment, like slaves, in order to swell the institution's finances [53]. Not long after, in October 1886, Allen left the asylum, unhappy and disillusioned.

Much of the history of the racist and autocratic cruelty of the model of 'moral treatment' that he instituted in the asylum was not written down, although we do have an oral history within the hospital. Allen's 'moral treatment' may have created a paternalistic mini-society within the asylum's walls in the 1870s, but this disappeared within a few short years of his departure in 1886, as the racist foundations on which it was constructed could not support its healthy continuance. My close study of the 1873 Jamaican Lunatic Asylum Law (later renamed the Mental Hospital Law) taught me an important lesson about the practical application of colonial governance of the time. The Colonial Governor ruled with an iron hand and social control was effected through the Chief Justice who controlled the judiciary, the police force, and the prisons; and the Senior Medical Officer of the Lunatic Asylum. The Senior Medical Officer (*aka* Physician Superintendent), under the 1873 Law, had awesome powers of detention and control over Jamaican people of all classes and walks of life. Between these three officers of the colonial state ruled from Whitehall in London, a system of absolute control of the society was maintained. It is only with this 'overstanding' (Rastafarian neologistic word meaning 'insight,' antithetically opposed to 'understanding' meaning 'knowledge') that the struggle between Allen and Grant after the Morant Bay Rebellion makes any psychohistorical sense. Allen was Eyre's man. Eyre ruled Jamaica with an 'iron fist' and was the chief catalyst of the Rebellion [46]. Allen's racist authoritarian practices were facilitated and encouraged by his immediate superior—Eyre. This relationship changed when Grant was sent by a colonial Whitehall to appease and ameliorate Jamaican society following the Rebellion and its aftermath. Allen's early political support in Jamaica diminished after Eyre departed following the Morant Bay debacle [39: 228, fn 68].

Not long after, in October 1886, Allen left the asylum, returned to England, and was dead within a few months. The principles and practices of 'moral management,' with their clear parallels to a 'civilizing' process, contrasted noticeably with the disparaging attitudes toward 'the Jamaican Negro' that he periodically espoused. I experienced at first hand the racist construction of the colonial lunatic asylum when I joined the staff of Bellevue Hospital in 1973 and was instrumental in helping to abolish the dualistic rich/poor, White/Black private ward social dichotomy that had existed there since its inception in 1861. Like most phenomena of history, if events are not written down and carefully recorded, then many can insist in future times that they had not transpired. And even then, they can easily be distorted to serve one perspective or another.

Toward a New Paradigm of the History of Madness

From the perspective of the Black agricultural workers who had to endure the vicissitudes of the Jamaica Lunatic Asylum, the construct of 'moral treatment' was just another authoritarian restraint mechanism used by the European ruling class to dress up or disguise the public policy issues of enslavement and the rapacious entrapment of their labor within this newly created colonial custodial institution. The moral treatment approach to mental disorder ostensibly based on humane psychosocial care or moral discipline that emerged in Europe in the late eighteenth century did not fare well in post-slavery societies like Jamaica. In fact, given the vastly different approaches to treating Jamaica's White and Brown inhabitants, it turned out to be merely an extension of the brutish plantation system, applied patronizingly to a disrespected Black population that had only recently been reluctantly released from chattel slavery by a ruthlessly dominant master class which still controlled the commanding heights of the economy. In this context, moral treatment was a glorified method of entrenching the master/servant relationship fostered by agents of a rampaging British ruling class that was intent on world domination and on finding ways to oppressively keep the rebellious colonized social dissenters under control. This was part of the purportedly sophisticated 'civilizing mission' and involved the ruthless institution of a system of control of, and acceptance by, people who were in a life and death struggle against this form of social entrapment. Christienna Fryar's [54] analysis of the British imperial scandal concerning the treatment of patients in the Jamaica Lunatic Asylum suggested that at the heart of the scandal was a debate about whether standards of treatment developed in Britain—symbolized by the image of the ideal asylum and the ideology of moral management—could and should be implemented in colonies. This debate was all the more fraught because the designation of moral management as the official protocol was recent, its implementation incomplete, and its underlying ideas contested. Britain's 'civilizing mission', that Smith [39] sees as seeking to promote both the 'custody' and the 'cure' of mentally disordered people, and an important element in the development of institutions for the insane, seems more of a fiction of arrogant British colonial brutishness than benevolent altruism. Smith's description of the ostensibly benign approach of the British toward provision for the colonial insane being reflected in the gradual permeation of the organizational framework that became known as 'moral management' has been challenged by the realities of the postcolonial scandal concerning the treatment of patients in the Jamaica Lunatic Asylum. The idea that 'moral treatment' at the asylum encompassed both custodial and curative aspects, providing structure, order, and discipline in the institution, while also encompassing interactions and activities geared toward promoting patients' recovery and rehabilitation, must be seen in my view as an absurd melange of the European paternalistic psychotic delusions. Fryar concludes that the idea of 'moral treatment helping to bolster the farcical concoction of the concept of moral management promulgated in postcolonial Britain' was essentially unstable.

The Later Colonial Period: Circa 1900–1960

To my knowledge, there are only three published journal articles written by Caribbean psychiatrists on the history of psychiatry in the Caribbean, two written by Michael Beaubrun [55, 56] and one by me [57]. These articles tend to focus primarily on the institutions and public policy surrounding the treatment of the mentally ill rather than a discourse to comprehend the clinical presentation and the origin and etiology of Caribbean peoples' abnormal behavior. The colonial government's thrust to provide mental health care through a chain of asylums across the region was met with the challenge from traditional healers to provide healing for the masses of the Caribbean people. In the immediate post-emancipation period, the doctors who delivered psychiatric care through the paradigm of the lunatic asylum were all White and predominantly European born. With the advent of emancipation, more Black people had the opportunity for education and attainment of professional medical status. The building of the Lunatic Asylum and the passage of the Lunatic Asylum Laws of 1862 and 1873 set the stage for the politicizing of the mentally ill in Jamaica and provided a platform for locking up political dissidents who challenged the legitimacy of colonialism. The nineteenth-century political struggles were rooted in Ethiopianism. The term Ethiopianism derived from its occurrence in the Bible (where Ethiopia is also referred to as Kush or Cush), especially Psalm 68:31, which states, 'let Ethiopia hasten to stretch out its hands to God' [58].

Ethiopianism propelled the revolutionary vision of the twentieth century. Case studies of political dissidents such as Alexander Bedward in 1895 provide hard evidence that the Jamaican colonial state used the Lunatic Asylum and the Lunatic Asylum Laws to muzzle political dissent [59]. Bedward was a political activist, religious prophet, and shepherd/missionary who had a huge following in August Town and across Jamaica. He preached a message of freedom and repatriation to Africa for Jamaican people. One afternoon when we were rehearsing the pageant *Madnificent Irations* we literally stumbled upon some very old clinical record ledgers of the mental hospital that were being dumped in the garbage during a nursing administration 'spring cleaning.' These documents were the original clinical records of Bedward and contained all the newspaper clippings of the time related to his arrest and incarceration. They showed that Bedward was initially arrested by the British government on the grounds that his revolutionary religious activism constituted treason; after the charges were withdrawn in 1895 he was incarcerated in the asylum.

Bedward developed a huge following in Jamaica as a leader demanding reparations as well as repatriation for the descendants of Africans enslaved in Jamaica; many myths and songs celebrated this folk hero. The Lunatic Asylum Laws, in conjunction with the anti-Obeah Law, led to the suppression of traditional communal healing and treatment systems. In fact, tertiary mental health care in Jamaica, through the establishment of the asylum and passage of the relevant legislation, also engaged in the practice of incarcerating members of the Rastafari movement between the 1930s and 1960s. Leonard Howell, generally regarded as the originator of the Rastafari movement, and who established the first Rastafarian commune at Pinnacle in St. Catherine, became a target of police raids in the 1930s and 1940s. An irritant to the colonial government, he was incarcerated in the asylum (renamed the Bellevue Hospital in 1946) and a police raid eventually destroyed his commune in 1958 [60]. There is mounting recorded evidence that confirms that the British colonial government used the legal structure and mental health institutions in the Caribbean to suppress political dissent and to stifle cultural and religious expression [61].

The struggle for psychiatry in the Caribbean became clearer in the period 1900–1960. The emergence of Black doctors and psychiatrists in the mental hospitals of the Caribbean began in 1915, all of whom were trained in North America or the UK. As mentioned in the previous chapter, my granduncle Dr. Hopetoun E. Bond (1879–1939), was the first Black psychiatrist in the Caribbean, practicing in Jamaica at the asylum between 1914 and 1919. He was followed by a trickle of foreign-trained Jamaican psychiatrists, which swelled into a stream of Jamaican-trained psychiatrists with the establishment of the University of the West Indies in 1948 and a Department of Psychiatry at that University in 1965.

In an attempt to reduce the stigma attached to regional asylums, the term 'Lunatic Asylum' was removed from institutional names in Barbados (Black Rock, 1905), Trinidad (St. Ann's, 1935), Jamaica (Bellevue, 1946) and Belize (Seaview, 1964). Although custodialization remained the main therapeutic principle, European treatment systems were embraced, including electroconvulsive therapy, insulin coma, early-stage social work, and occupational therapy. Consequently, as the mental hospital grew in importance, so the nidus of stigma attached to mental illness, overcrowding, and institutionalization burgeoned in the wider society. This was paralleled by the development of Obeah and other traditional healing systems in all Caribbean territories [62].

Notes

1. Wilson J (September 14, 1742–August 21, 1798), was one of the Founding Fathers of the United States and a signatory of the United States Declaration of Independence.
2. Sherman R (April 19, 1721–July 23, 1793) was an early American lawyer and politician, as well as a Founding Father of the United States.

Bibliography

1. Hickling FW (1985) Poem "Westminster System" (Unpublished).
2. Cartwright SA (May 1851) Report on the Diseases and Physical Peculiarities of the Negro Race. *The New Orleans Medical and Surgical Journal*, 691–715.
3. Jackson V (2003) An Early History—African American Mental Health. In *Our In Own Voice: African American Stories of Oppression, Survival and Recovery in the Mental Health System*, pp. 1–36, 48. Published by author. https://power2u.org/in-our-own-voice-african-american-stories-of-oppression-survival-and-recovery-in-mental-health-systems-by-vanessa-jackson/.
4. De las Casas B (1992) [E Book #20321] *A Short Account of the Destruction of the Indies. Project Gutenberg, p. 23*, written 1542, published 1552. Nigel Griffin, ed. London: Penguin.
5. Duff C (1936) *The Truth About Columbus and the Discovery of America.* New York: Random House.
6. Hickling FW (2009) The European American Psychosis: A Psychohistoriographic Perspective of Contemporary Western Civilization. *The Journal of Psychohistory. A Publication of the Institute for Psychohistory, 37*(1), 67–81.
7. Hickling FW (2007) *Psychohistoriography: A Postcolonial Psychoanalytic and Psychotherapeutic Model.* University of the West Indies, Mona, CARIMENSA Press.
8. Three-Fifths Compromise. http://en.wikipedia.org/wiki/Three-Fifths_Compromise.
9. Cahill K (2011) Who Owns the World? *New Statesman*, March 14.

10. Cundall F, Pietersz JL (1919) The Abbot of Jamaica to the King of Spain July 1611. In *Jamaica Under the Spaniards, Abstracted from the Archives of Seville.* Institute of Jamaica, pp. 34–35.
11. Minority Rights Group International (2007) *World Directory of Minorities and Indigenous Peoples—Trinidad and Tobago.* Available at: https://www.refworld.org/docid/4954ce55c.html, accessed 24 March 2020.
12. Hitchens C (2010) *Hitch 22: A Memoir: Some Confessions and Contradictions.* New York, Boston: McClelland & Stewart.
13. Williams E (1944 [1970]) *Capitalism and Slavery.* USA: University of North Carolina Press; London: Longmans.
14. Lindqvist S (1992) *"Exterminate All the Brutes": One Man's Odyssey into the Heart of Darkness and the Origins of European Genocide.* Translated from the Swedish by Joan Tate. New York, London: The New Press, pp. 173–174.
15. Carew J (1994) *The Rape of Paradise: Columbus and the Birth of Racism in America.* New York: A & B Publishers, pp. 264–266.
16. Final Call (2009) Willie Lynch letter: The Making of a Slave. http://www.finalcall.com/artman/publish/Perspectives_1/Willie_Lynch_letter_The_Making_of_a_Slave.shtml.
17. Rosenzweig R (2001) The Road to Xanadu: Public and Private Pathways on the History Web. *The Journal of American, History, 88*(2), 548–579.
18. Cobb, WJ (2004) *Is Willie Lynch's Letter Real?* Jim Crow Museum of Racist Memorabilia, Ferris State University.
19. Patterson O (1967) *The Sociology of Slavery: An Analysis of the Origins, Development and Structure of Negro Slave Society in Jamaica.* London: McGibbon & Kee Ltd., p. 82.
20. Halliday A (1828) *A General View of the Present State of Lunatics and Lunatic Asylums in Great Britain, Ireland, and Some Other Kingdoms.* London: Thomas and George Underwood, pp. 79–80.
21. Lester D (1998) Suicidal Behavior in African-American Slaves. *OMEGA—Journal of Death and Dying, 37*(1), 1–13. https://doi.org/10.2190/qx9p-68dp-hx8u-l4aa.
22. Hickling FW (1988) Psychiatry in the Commonwealth Caribbean: A Brief Historical Overview. *Psychiatric Bulletin, 12*, 434–436.
23. Patterson O (1967) Select Committee on Slave Trade 1790–1791. Quoted from *The Sociology of Slavery: An Analysis of the Origins, Development and Structure of Negro Slave Society in Jamaica.* London: McGibbon and Kee.
24. Blassingame JW (Ed.) (1977) *Slave Testimony.* Baton Rouge, LA: Louisiana State University.
25. Paton D (2001) Punishment, Crime, and the Bodies of Slaves in Eighteenth-Century Jamaica. *Journal of Social History, 34*(4), 923–954.
26. Day TR (2016) *Jamaican Revolts in British Press and Politics, 1760–1825.* Virginia Commonwealth University. https://scholarscompass.vcu.edu/etd/4089.

27. Nettleford RM (1978) *Caribbean Cultural Identity: The Case Study of Jamaica*. Kingston: Institute of Jamaica, p. 18.
28. Hickling FW (2001) The Cyclical Pattern of Violent Rebellion in Jamaica 1660 to 1999. In *The International Conference on Crime and Criminal Justice in the Caribbean*, Hosted by the Department of Government of the University of the West Indies.
29. Associated Press (1999) Protests Over Rise in Fuel Tax Disrupt Streets in Jamaica. *The New York Times*, April 22.
30. Cook A, Spinazzola J, Ford J, Lanktree C, Blaustein M, Cloitre M, Hubbard R, Kagan R, Liautaud J, Mallah K, Olafson E, van der Kolk B (2005) Complex Trauma in Children and Adolescents. *Psychiatric Annals, 35*(5), 390–398.
31. Conolly J (1847) *On the Construction and Government of Lunatic Asylums*, ed. R Hunter, I MacAlpine (reprint 1968). London, pp. 65–66. Google Scholar.
32. Bowerbank LQ (1858) *A Circular Letter;* J. Scott, *A Reply to a Letter by Lewis Quier Bowerbank....to the Commissioners of the Public Hospital and Lunatic Asylum of Kingston, Jamaica, Relative to the Present State and Management of These Institutions* (Kingston, Jamaica: Jordon and Osborn).
33. Pratt A (1860) *Seven Months in the Kingston Lunatic Asylum, and What I Saw There* (Kingston: George Henderson, Savage, & Co.); *Official Documents on the Case of Ann Pratt, the Reputed Authoress of a Certain Pamphlet, Entitled 'Seven Months in the Kingston Lunatic Asylum, and What I Saw There'* (Kingston, Jamaica: Jordon and Osborn, 1860).
34. Rouse R (1860) *New Light on Dark Deeds; Being Jottings from the Diary of Richard Rouse, Late Warden of the Lunatic Asylum of Kingston, Edited by his son*. Kingston, Jamaica: Gall and Myers.
35. Jones M (2008) "The Most Cruel and Revolting Crimes": The Treatment of the Mentally Ill in Mid-Nineteenth Century Jamaica. *Journal of Caribbean History, 42*(2), 290–309.
36. *The Lancet*, 23 October, 25 December 1858, 26 March, 6 August, 3 September, 16 December 1859, 4 August, 17 December 1860, 26 January 1861.
37. *The Times*, 30 August, 1 September, 8 September 1859.
38. Smith L (2010) Caribbean Bedlam: The Development of the Lunatic Asylum System in Britain's West Indian Colonies 1838–1914. *Journal of Caribbean History, 44*(1), 1–47.
39. Smith L (2014) *Insanity, Race and Colonialism: Managing Mental Disorder in the Post-Emancipation British Caribbean, 1838–1914*. Basingstoke, UK: Palgrave Macmillan.
40. Waddell HM (1863) *Twenty-Nine Years in the West Indies and Central Africa: A Review of Missionary Work and Adventure 1829–1858*. Harvard University; London and New York: T. Nelson and Sons. https://archive.org/details/twentynineyears00waddgoog/page/n29/mode/2up.

41. Foucault M (1971) *Madness and Civilization: A History of Insanity in the Age of Reason.* London: Tavistock.
42. Lakritz K (2009) Michel Foucault's Madness and Civilization: A History of Insanity in the Age of Reason. *Psychiatric Times, 26*(6), 45. Accessed 25 March 2020.
43. France A (1894) *Le Lys Rouge* [The Red Lily] ch. 7 Paris: Calmann-Lévy.
44. *Jamaica Gleaner*, 3 November 1869.
45. Evans JF (2005) *Edward Eyre, Race and Colonial Governance.* Dunedin: Otago University Press, pp. 113–143.
46. Dutton G (1967) *The Hero as Murderer: The Life of Edward John Eyre, Australian Explorer and Governor of Jamaica, 1815–1901.* London: William Collins.
47. Moore BL, Johnson MA (2004) *Neither Led Nor Driven; Contesting British Cultural Imperialism, 1865–1920.* Mona, Jamaica: University of West Indies Press, pp. 1–6.
48. TNA, CO 137/477, 18 July 1874, Allen to Colonial Secretary, fo.196.
49. Barbados National Archives, PAM C 72, Report of the Commission on Poor Relief, 1875–77, Appendix, Report of Thomas Allen, M.D., Medical Superintendent and Director of the Jamaica Lunatic Asylum, to His Excellency the Governor of Barbados. Copy also in TNA CO 31/67, Minutes of Proceedings of Barbados House of Assembly, 1875–6, Appendix D.
50. *Jamaica Gleaner*, 12 August, 17 November 1880, 13 September 1883.
51. TNA CO 140/186, Annual Report of the Jamaica Lunatic Asylum, for the year ended 30th September 1883, pp. 165–166.
52. *Jamaica Gleaner*, 13 June 1885.
53. *Jamaica Gleaner*, 22 September 1886.
54. Fryar CD (2016) Imperfect Models: The Kingston Lunatic Asylum Scandal and the Problem of Postemancipation Imperialism. *Journal of British Studies, 55*(4), 709–727. https://doi.org/10.1017/jbr.2016.70.
55. Beaubrun MH, Bannister PY, Lewis L, et al. (1976) The History of Psychiatry in the West Indies. In G. Howells (Ed.), *History of World Psychiatry.* New York: Brunner/Mazel.
56. Beaubrun MH (1992) Caribbean Psychiatry Yesterday, Today and Tomorrow. *History of Psychiatry, 3*(11), 371–382.
57. Hickling FW (2009) The High Cost of Poverty: Mental Health Perspectives from the Caribbean Diaspora. *International Psychiatry, 6*(2), 29–30.
58. Melissa Petruzzello and the Editors of Encyclopaedia Britannica (2017) Ethiopianism—African Religion. https://www.britannica.com/topic/Ethiopianism.
59. Hickling FW, Gibson RC (2005) The History of Caribbean Psychiatry. In FW Hickling, E Sorel (Eds.), *Images of Psychiatry: The Caribbean.* Kingston, Jamaica: Department of Community Health and Psychiatry, University of the West Indies, Mona.

60. Dagnini JK (2009) Rastafari: Alternative Religion and Resistance against "White" Christianity. *Études caribéennes*, April 2009. Retrieved 14 March 2012. http://etudescaribeennes.revues.org/3665. https://doi.org/10.4000/etudescaribeennes.3665.
61. Tinker H (1974) *A New System of Slavery: The Export of Indian Labour Overseas 1830–1920*. London: Oxford University Press.
62. Hickling FW, James C (2005) Traditional Mental Health Practices in Jamaica: On the Phenomenology of Red Eye, Bad Mind and Obeah. In FW Hickling, E Sorel (Eds.), *Images of Psychiatry: The Caribbean*. Kingston, Jamaica: Department of Community Health and Psychiatry, University of the West Indies, Mona.

CHAPTER 3

The Challenge to the Mental Health Ideology of the Colonizer

He left Elizabeth the Monarch
Sitting smiling on her throne
To overlook our business
While starving Black man groan. [1]

Common histories of colonialism and slavery in the New World pose the question of whether there is a living legacy that has been derived from European colonialism and transatlantic African slavery. We who are descendants of Africans enslaved in the New World have grown up with a grotesque concept of self and a distorted concept of freedom. Our warped concepts of freedom have emerged following emancipation, manumission, or colonial independence; legal impositions that have emerged from the reality of forced enslavement or compulsory colonization by greedy, sociopathic slave owners and colonizers. The European urge to own and dominate the people and property of the rest of the world attained obsessional intensity, and no doubt has been the single most causative factor of mental pathology in human history. Slavery and the trafficking of slaves were shameful aspects of the involvement of Europe in the New World. Robin Blackburn [2] defined the slave status and condition as a purely social construction—that of a social isolate, an outsider, a person without kin, a person subject to the complete and arbitrary authority of the master, a person who could be whipped or tortured or sexually abused, a piece of property, and by virtue of the foregoing, an instrument. The very enumeration of such qualities must remind

F. W. Hickling, *Decolonization of Psychiatry in Jamaica*,
https://doi.org/10.1007/978-3-030-48489-7_3

us that slavery was not a suprahistorical essence but has to be produced and perpetuated, enlisting the support of the free population and adapting the slave to the particular use required.

Manumission, 'the formal emancipation from slavery' [3] is the act of a slave owner freeing his or her slaves. Different approaches developed, each specific to the time and place of a society's slave system. The motivations of slave owners in manumitting slaves were complex and varied [4]. Manumission is a juridical action in which property rights were surrendered, and in which the former slave assumed a new legal personality and new legal responsibility [5]. All definitions of the process of emancipation from slavery imply explicitly or implicitly that the freedom attained derives from the legal release by the slave owner. The process dictated a wide spectrum of freed persons—completely freed, partially freed with contractual obligation to the ex-master, partial self-purchased, tenants, and peons. Sociologist Mee-Yan Cheung-Judge [6] observed that although objectively and technically freed by their masters, in fact many aspects of the lives of the freed person either remained the same or grew worse, and that from the seventeenth to the nineteenth century, manumission occurred in most parts of the New World. For freed persons, though significantly better off than slaves, life was often more brutal, and they suffered considerable social, educational, and religious restrictions.

Evidence from the Spanish, Dutch, French, and British Caribbean indicates that status inconsistencies and social prejudices were especially brutal. Once freed, Blacks remained at the bottom of the social order, subject to physical and verbal abuse. This glaring discrepancy between expectation and reality in their legal, social, political, educational, and religious rights was often bitterly resented by the freed persons and had substantial impact on their self-perceptions, identity structure, interpersonal relations and their social and communal life [7]. The first contemporary Caribbean psychiatrist to challenge the pathological psychosociological concepts of freedom of descendants of Africans enslaved in the New World was Martinique-born psychiatrist Frantz Fanon, miscegenated son of descendants of African slaves of the French Caribbean, whose profound work and writings of the psychology of slavery and colonialism in France and Algeria have shaken and enriched the world. Born in Fort-de-France, Martinique in 1925, he fought for the Free French during World War II, and studied medicine and psychiatry in Paris. His early psychiatric career was spent in the Blida-Joinville Mental

Hospital in Algeria in 1953 and he worked there until he resigned in 1956 to devote himself to the cause of Algerian independence.

His pioneering work [7, 8] has helped us to focus on the reality that mental health cannot be achieved without viewing the relationship of the individual to oppression in repressive socioeconomic and political conditions. Fanon, although born in Martinique, never practiced psychiatry in the Caribbean. However, his origin in post-slavery Caribbean society no doubt helped to catalyze his insistence that psychotherapeutic forms must include methodologies to challenge the psychopathology of racism in the context of decolonization. Fanon contended that colonialism breeds psychopathology and its own form of madness in both the colonizer and the colonized. The Pan-Africanist ideas promoted by Jamaican Marcus Garvey [9] and Trinidadian George Padmore [10] during the first decades of the twentieth century have been crucial to the mental health of Black people around the world. The self-assertion of Black people and the rejection of White institutionalized racism were the main thrust of Garvey's and Padmore's message, and fuelled a revolution of political and cultural transformation of Black people across the Caribbean, the Americas, and Africa. This message was picked up and articulated in a most emphatic way by Fanon in his revolutionary work *The Wretched of the Earth* (1961). He articulated the need for psychiatry worldwide to see itself in dialectical constructs and paradigms. He rejected Eurocentric bourgeois concepts of madness and their limited methodologies for treating the casualties of the system that they had created. The underpinnings of cultural therapy articulated in *Madnificent Irations* are clearly derived from the Pan-Africanism of Garvey and Padmore and the psycho-political analysis enunciated by Fanon. Although Fanon is best known from his four books on the psychopathology induced by colonization, *Black Skin, White Masks* (1952), *A Dying Colonialism* (1959), the much more well-known *The Wretched of the Earth*, and a posthumous publication of his writings, *Toward the African Revolution* (1964), the many psychiatric publications that he wrote between 1951 and 1960 are infrequently studied. However, Fanon always saw himself as a psychiatrist first and rarely stopped practicing, whether in France, Algeria, or Tunisia [11]. Jean Khalfa, a philosopher, linguist and senior lecturer at Trinity College, Cambridge, has helped to illustrate Fanon's contribution as a psychiatrist to consider the essential role of culture in mental illness, and finally to create an institution of psychiatric care outside of the asylum which he saw as a blueprint for mental health care in the future. Fanon was the first Caribbean psychiatrist to identify mental illness as a product of colonialism and emancipation. In one of his lesser known publications, he describes mental illness as a 'true pathology of freedom.'

There is extensive documentation of the colonial history of exploitation of the Caribbean as part of the European appetite for conquest and settlement and the ruthless, socially engineered European imposition of African slavery in the New World [12]. Indigenous peoples in North and South America and in Australia, New Zealand, and the Southern Pacific attempting to resist the European invasion were ruthlessly destroyed, and unparalleled acts of human cruelty and exploitation saw the European development of African slavery to meet the insatiable hunger of the colonizers for wealth and profit from colonial plantations of exploitation and plunder. There is little doubt that the complex traumas of genocide and slavery perpetrated by the European colonizers were the progenitors of the racism and economic exploitation which are manifest worldwide today. The question to be answered is whether *slavery and emancipation* were the aetiologic precursors of contemporary mental illness, in both Blacks and Whites. European colonization and exploitation engendered violent struggles for freedom in every continent. Violent struggles culminating in homicide and suicide were the major manifestations of mental health pathology from the sixteenth to the eighteenth century. Genocide and slavery, which were practiced routinely, were abandoned by the European colonizers only after the intensification of the violent struggles of the colonized and enslaved peoples had made military containment by the colonizer simply too expensive to maintain.

A comprehensive study of the effects of this imposition on the inhabitants of Caribbean territories began to emerge in the mid-twentieth century. While working with the West Indian Social Survey in Jamaica (1947–1949), British social psychologist Madeline Kerr conducted a seminal anthropological study of conflict and personality development in Jamaica [13]. Her work encapsulates historical perspectives of cultural tensions stemming from the paradoxical juxtaposition between African heritage and values, and the imposition of Western (British) attitudes and values that arose during slavery. She identified that these two conflicting cultural ideologies have left Jamaicans 'bewildered and insecure,' suggesting that the people of this new culture can only be psychologically free by somehow having to shake off the bitterness of the past, while at the same time admitting that the past and to some extent the present have left very deep scars [13].

My first sight of Africa, my motherland, was profound and emotional. I was a fledgling consultant psychiatrist working in the Bellevue Hospital in Jamaica. My first visit to mother Africa in 1979 brought me face to face with Fanon's magnificence, when I attended the Frantz Fanon International Conference in Mogadishu, Somalia. This was a historic conference honoring his inspirational work. At that conference, I met for the first time Black psychologists and educators from around the world. My first glimpse of Fanon as a Caribbean psychiatrist came at this conference. Fanon's work and teachings were not part of the British colonial psychiatric practice, which was the foundation of my professional training. The guiding navigational lighthouse in my half century of psychiatric practice has been Fanon's core teaching that psychiatric understanding is incomplete and invalid without the consideration of political oppression and exploitation. Fanon's seminal works, although infrequently referenced in Anglophone psychiatric and medical circles, are well known in social studies and have been a shining beacon for a few Third World psychiatrists.

It is not a coincidence that the contemporary call to psychologi cal determination of the effects of slavery on the sociopsychology of descendants of Africans enslaved in the New World is coming from the Caribbean islands of Martinique and Guadeloupe. My most profound encounter with Fanon's profound 'overstanding' came nearly forty years later when I attended the a conference in November 2016 titled 'Colloque Scientifique International L'esclavage: quel impact sur la psychologie des populations? (Slavery: what is its impact on the psychology of populations?)' as part of the United Nations' International Decade for people of African Descent, 2015–2024. After I had made my presentation at this conference [14], which outlined the postcolonial metamorphosis in mental health delivery that we have achieved in Jamaica since independence in 1962, many psychiatrists and sociologists in attendance commented to me how my work in Jamaica paralleled Fanon's work as a psychiatrist. Armed with this new personal insight into Fanon the psychiatrist as opposed to Fanon the sociologist and political revolutionary, I embarked on a personal rediscovery of his writings and work in psychiatry. I realized that his writings outside of his translated books were all in French and would have escaped my limited Anglophone worldview.

In the process I learned how rooted his insights were in biological psychiatry and how his experiences propelled him from psychoanalysis into social psychiatry.

As I read Khalfa's interpretation of Fanon's writing as a psychiatrist I reflected that Fanon's seminal contribution to medicine and psychiatry involved his clear delineation of phenomenology from neurology and his profound insight of the phenomenological context in the social space, and how that complexity connected to the awesome simplicity of psychosocial therapy. He declared that mental illness presents itself as a true *pathology of freedom*, with the disease situating the ill person in a world where his freedom, his will, his desires are constantly broken by obsessions, inhibitions, counter-orders, anxieties. The classic hospitalization limits the patient's field of action, forbids any compensation, and restricts him to the closed field of the hospital, ordering him to exorcise the unreal world of fantasy [15].

It is fitting that Charles-Nicolas Aimé, Professor of Psychiatry in Martinique and President of the Association Régionale 'FIRST CARAÏBES', chose to commemorate Fanon's legacy to the birthplace they shared. He asked the conference attendees to focus on the psychotraumatic consequences, common denominators and protective factors of psyches shaped by slavery. He emphasised that at this, the first scientific event to specifically address the psychological consequences of slavery, the challenge was also to tackle the linkages between slavery, alienation, and internalized racism, taking on board that the slave trade exclusively concerned Black people and that from the sixteenth century, slavery changed both in nature and in scale. This has led to a racialized and layered vision of humanity that has taken a particularly heavy toll on the Caribbean, with its present day population descended from 10 million deported Africans [16].

The conference brought together neuroscientists, sociologists, psychologists, psychiatrists, writers, and artists from Europe and North America, each of whom contributed a report on the sequelae of slavery among our patients. I was the only psychiatrist from the English-speaking Caribbean invited to contribute to the discourse. The challenge for me was to get to the conference in Martinique from my home in Jamaica. I was informed by my travel agent that I needed a Schengen visa to enter Martinique, which is a Department of France. The French Embassy in Jamaica informed me that it was unable to issue the visa for me to enter Martinique, and that to secure the visa I had to fly to Panama City and apply to the Embassy there for the required document. This would require me to stay in a hotel for one week while the visa was being processed. The visa having been issued, I would then have to return to Jamaica as I could only enter Martinique on that visa by flying from Kingston. Thus, for a Jamaican, with a Jamaican passport, a short flight of 1777 km (1104 miles) between the two Caribbean islands could only be achieved by an additional flight of 2042 km and an additional expenditure of airfare to Panama and a one week hotel bill. This illustrated the madness of the present-day postcolonial Caribbean. The Caribbean islands are still owned if not controlled by the six European nations who colonized the New World. Europe has been able to secure the Caribbean islands as a vacation paradise for Europeans, secured in these postcolonial times without the expense and headache of governance. The freedom of the citizens who live in those islands is patently not free. The delusion of freedom for Caribbean Black people is a reality.

The revolution in transcultural psychiatric thinking and research brought about by Fanon's work has profoundly challenged European psychiatric discernment, setting the stage for similar explorations in the Caribbean. These insights have straddled the plethora of anthropological and sociological research findings that have emerged in the Caribbean on contemporary psychopathology of people of color. There are many dimensions in contemporary Britain in which inequalities in mental health care are evident. Jamaican-born sociologist, cultural theorist and political activist Stuart Hall [17] has described the social conditions in Britain as a manifestation of internal colonialism and suggests that migrants to Britain have not been allowed to participate in equitable social and economic development in that country. Although African Caribbean people have made significant contributions to the development and prosperity of Britain in the past four hundred years, they have not received their rightful share of its wealth and social benefit provisions. Many epidemiological studies in the past three decades have confirmed the racist experiences endured by African Caribbean people in England. Epidemiological studies of mental illness in the Caribbean point to potent and complex environmental and psychosocial stresses that trigger this condition in migrants from the Caribbean to Europe. Since the demise of the European colonial empires, there has been a profound migration of large swathes of postcolonial peoples to the homelands of the colonizers. The direction of migration has been strongly influenced by previous colonial ties. Migration to Britain from the English-speaking Caribbean since World War II has been extraordinarily high, particularly by those who have been educated to tertiary level [18]. As I write, I mourn the passing of my UWI medical school batchmate Dr. Franklyn Jacobs, who established his own general practice in 1982, working predominantly with the Greek community in North London. As I do so, I reflect on the thousands of African Caribbean doctors, nurses and other health professionals who have also contributed so much to the NHS. Born in St. Vincent, Franklyn was, with David (later Lord) Pitt and Eddie Simon, a co-founder of the African Caribbean Medical Society. Knowledge of the mental health implications of migration are essential in the armamentarium of the contemporary mental health professional from the perspective of making the diagnosis in people from a variety of ethnic and cultural backgrounds, and understanding the pitfalls of clinical and cultural competences that can occur especially for practitioners from the dominant host migrant countries, where prejudice and cultural misinterpretations can be protean. My experience as a Black Jamaican consultant psychiatrist in England provides the crucible for this case study examination of mental illness in African Caribbeans in the UK. At the time of writing, as the country gears up to cope with the urgent demands of Brexit, and xenophobic and myopic cultural formulations continue to be challenged, there is a need for cultural humility and insight on the part of practicing clinicians, in order to provide appropriate levels of mental health care for the individuals, families, and communities that comprise the multi-ethnic society of modern-day Britain.

I first learned of the anti-psychiatry movement in Britain while a psychiatric resident of the University of Edinburgh in 1973, when I heard a lecture given by Scottish psychiatrist R.D. Laing, who was considered to be its founder. His lecture introduced me to the ideas of Jacques Lacan, David Cooper, and Thomas Szasz, the prominent writers of the time who challenged accepted ways of understanding the psychotic experience. Based on Marxist theory, Laing's ideas rejected the illness model of psychiatry, advocating the intelligibility of the psychotic experience, and the conviction that the understanding of madness must be based on the study of the family [19]. I was subsequently fascinated by the work of Szasz [20] and his rejection of the essence of psychiatric morbidity. Mervat Nasser [19] suggests that while the tendency among psychiatrists is to regard the anti-psychiatry movement as having entered the annals of modern psychiatric history and to look back on its ideology as an attempt to flirt with polemics at the expense of scientific thought and enquiry, it would be naive to assume that it has had little or no impact on the conventional practice of psychiatry. She suggests that the development of advocacy groups such as the UK organization MIND, which are concerned with the legal, social and personal conditions of people receiving treatment, has profoundly restrained the power of psychiatry. Nasser further suggests that the development of community centers for the treatment of mental illness and the distancing from the 'medical model' is perhaps the most profound legacy of the anti-psychiatry movement.

There is no doubt that my own psychiatric thinking and development has been powerfully influenced by the Edinburgh school of psychiatry. David Henderson mentored the Grenadian/Trinidadian Professor of Psychiatry Michael Beaubrun at the University of the West Indies, who taught us how to treat acute psychosis in the general medical wards of medical hospitals [21]. Morris Carstairs at the Royal Edinburgh Hospital nurtured a group of young psychiatrists and psychologists, called the 'Carstairs babies', that included Tim Harding, Sashi Sashidharan, Raymond Cochrane, Isam Babiker, Rustam (Rusty) Framrose, and many others, who have been successful in promulgating the community treatment message of Carstairs. A number of Caribbean colleagues including Janet LaGrenade, Franklin Ottey, and Trevor Lindsay benefited from Beaubrun's and Carstairs' mentoring. Morris Carstairs was a very unusual Brit. Born in India to a Scottish missionary father, at the time of the British Raj, he spent his childhood in India and was fluent in Hindi. Carstairs understood colonialism from within, and as Professor of Psychiatry and President (1968–1972) of the World Mental Health Organization, he diligently selected young psychiatric scholars from the British Commonwealth and organized scholarships for them to study with him at the University of Edinburgh. I have a vivid memory of attending a tutorial led by him, in which he gave his Commonwealth charges an assignment to write an essay plan for the reconstruction of the mental health services in their country. My essay appeared in the *Sunday Gleaner* on July 15, 1973, following my return to my homeland [22]. Titled 'A Plan for Psychiatry in Jamaica', it subsequently became a blueprint for the decolonization of the Jamaican mental health services.

As I further reflected on my own experience working as a consultant psychiatrist in Palmerston North in New Zealand in 1993, and at the Aston and Smallheath NHS practice in North Birmingham in the closing five years of the millennium, in the context of my previous 20 years' experience at the postcolonial Jamaican Bellevue Hospital, I began to conclude that the British and European anti-psychiatry movement could not make sense without the Fanon perspective on the brutal effects of European colonization. 'Therapeutic Community' and 'Community Engagement', fundamental tenets of my psychiatric thinking and practice that I developed while working in Jamaica and other former colonial territories, emerged in part from the anti-psychiatry movement in Britain. The formulation of the term 'European-American psychosis' emerged from the psychohistoriographic study pioneered at Bellevue. It posited the delusion of White supremacy (i.e. 'doing God's work') as the most likely explanation of the insanity of European-based psychiatry. It also reflected my experience of working at what had until recently been a colonial asylum. Only the drive for total domination can explain the murderous violence that a small core group of White people inflicted both on themselves and the peoples of the rest of the world. It included the slavery imposed on African people, the grotesque institutions of incarceration and custodialization, and the bizarre Procrustean[1] imposition, throughout the world, of a capitalist economic system. The emergence of psychohistoriographic cultural therapy as a methodology of dialectically and culturally challenging the European-American delusion is suggested to be an important anti-colonial and anti-psychiatry therapeutic construct.

Bibliography

1. Hickling FW (1985) Poem "Westminster System" (Unpublished).
2. Blackburn R (1988) Defining Slavery—Its Special Features and Social Role. In LJ Archer (Ed.), *Slavery and Other Forms of Unfree Labour*. London and New York: Routledge, p. 276.
3. Merriam-Webster. https://www.merriam-webster.com/dictionary/manumission.
4. Wikipedia. https://en.wikipedia.org/wiki/Manumission.
5. Schwartz SB (1974) The Manumission of Slaves in Colonial Brazil: Bahia 1684–1745. *Hispanic American Historical Review*, *54*, 603–635 (pp. 604–605).

[1]In Greek mythology, **Procrustes (Ancient Greek** Προκρούστης *Prokroustes*) or 'the stretcher [who hammers out the metal],' also known as **Prokoptas** or **Damastes** (Δαμαστής, "subduer"), was a rogue smith and bandit from Attica who attacked people by stretching them or cutting off their legs, so as to force them to fit the size of an iron bed. The word 'Procrustean' is thus used to describe situations where different lengths or sizes or properties are fitted to an arbitrary standard. Wikipedia, https://en.wikipedia.org/wiki/Procrustes.

6. Cheung-Judge LM-Y (1988) The Social-Psychological Analysis of Manumission. In LJ Archer (Ed.), *Slavery and Other Forms of Unfree Labour*. London and New York: Routledge, pp. 240–241.
7. Fanon F (1967) *The Wretched of the Earth*. London: Penguin Books.
8. Fanon F (1968) *Black Skin, White Masks*. New York: Grove.
9. Garvey AJ (1967) *The Philosophy and Opinions of Marcus Garvey, or Africa for the Africans*. London: Frank Cass.
10. Padmore G (1936) *How Britain Rules Africa*. London: Wishart Books.
11. Fanon, F (2018). *Alienation and Freedom*. Eds. J Khalfa, RC Young. Translated by S Corcoran. London: Bloomsbury Academic, pp. 1–7.
12. Williams E (1973) *From Columbus to Castro: The History of the Caribbean, 1492–1969*. London: Andre Deutsch.
13. Kerr M (1952) *Personality and Conflict in Jamaica*. London: Collins/ Sangster's, p. x.
14. Hickling FW (2018) *Shattering the Delusions of Slavery: Psychosocial Re-engineering of Postcolonial Jamaica*. Démanteler les délires de l'esclavage: vers ingénierie psychosociale en Jamaïque postcolonial. Eds. C-N Aimé & B Bowser, L'esclavage: quel impact sur la psychologie des populations? Paris.
15. Fanon F (1959) L'Hospitalisation de jour en psychiatrie: valeur et limites. *La Tunisie médicale, 37*(10), 689–732 (pp. 717, 723).
16. Aimé C-N (2016) Preamble. International Scientific Colloquium. Slavery: What Is Its Impact on the Psychology of Populations. http://ciphage.com/?lg=en.
17. Hall S (1992) New Ethnicities. In J Donald, A Rattansi (Eds.), *Race and Culture*. London: Sage.
18. Mishra P (2006) Emigration and Brain Drain: Evidence from the Caribbean. International Monetary Fund Working Paper. Retrieved from http://www.imf.org/external/pubs/ft/wp/2006/wp0625.pdf.
19. Nasser M (1995) The Rise and Fall of Anti-psychiatry. *Psychiatric Bulletin, 19*, 743–746.
20. Szasz T (1972) *The Myth of Mental Illness: Foundations of a Theory of Personal Conduct*. London: Granada Publishing.
21. Beaubrun MH (1968) A project for the West Indies (Chapter 21). In R Williams, L Ozarin (Eds.), *Community Mental Health, an International Perspective*. San Francisco: Jossey-Bass.
22. Hickling FW (1973) A Plan for Psychiatry in Jamaica. *Sunday Gleaner*, July 15.

CHAPTER 4

Madnificent Irations: What's in a Name?

Know that it is the same Westminster
That rules our little nation
Decimated Black man's culture
By building the plantation. [1]

On the evening of August 30, 1978, on the island of Jamaica in the central Caribbean, a pageant called *Madnificent Irations* had its opening performance. It was held in a unique, circular open-air performance center built of bamboo and called the Garden Theatre, situated in the grounds of the former Jamaica Lunatic Asylum, now Bellevue Hospital, built nearly 120 years earlier. Fifteen hundred people, headed by the nation's Governor-General, Florizel Glasspole, and a slew of government and other dignitaries saw a cast of fifty patients and staff from the mental hospital launch a three-and-a-half-hour long pageant depicting the history of madness in Jamaica and the history of the Lunatic Asylum in that country. Since that time the name *Madnificent Irations* has sounded in different parts of the world from Canada to the UK, at transcultural psychiatry conferences [2], and in psychiatric [3], postcolonial and entertainment journals as a unique signifier of cultural therapy: popular theatre and drama as therapy.

Madnificent Irations is a neologism. '…A neologism (/niːˈɒlədʒɪzəm/; from Greek νέο- *néo-*, "new" and λόγος *lógos*, "speech, utterance") is the name for a newly coined term, word, or phrase that may be in the process of entering common use, but that has not yet been accepted

F. W. Hickling, *Decolonization of Psychiatry in Jamaica*,
https://doi.org/10.1007/978-3-030-48489-7_4

into mainstream language. Neologisms are often directly attributable to a specific person, publication, period, or event…' [4]. They are often encountered in psychiatry, where they are used to describe words that have meaning only to the person who uses them, independent of their common meaning [5]. According to renowned German psychiatrist and phenomenologist Karl Jaspers, neologisms are employed by patients *intentionally* to describe feelings or things for which customary speech has not yet found words, and *unintentionally* while describing things during acute states; these usages then continue when their condition has become chronic [6]. Neologistic words and phrases have been found very commonly in the speech patterns of patients in the Bellevue Hospital and in Jamaican parlance. The phrase 'Madnificent Irations' was created intentionally to describe 'the magnificent dialectic thinking of descendants of Africans enslaved in the New World' with *madnificent* being neologistically inverted from the English word *magnificent* meaning 'extremely beautiful, elaborate, impressive or excellent' [7], and *irations* the Rastafarian neologism for creation. The word 'madnificent' was definitely and intentionally invented to replace magnificent, challenging in no uncertain terms who precisely is being described as mad: the colonial enslavers or the Africans enslaved in the New World!

The most important symbol of all cultural expressions is that of language. The imposition of European slavery and colonialism has significantly altered the speech patterns of the Jamaican people, and Afro-Caribbeans worldwide. Celebrated Jamaican poet Louise Bennett chose not to work in English, the official language of Jamaica, but in the language most Jamaicans speak. She explicitly defended the dignity and autonomy of the Jamaican Creole and asserted [8] that Europeans arrogantly and pompously claim English as a *derivation* of French, German, and other languages, but Jamaican Creole is a *corruption* of English. Bennett proclaimed that this pomposity was '*an unfairity*', asserting that the African ancestors of Jamaica choose to disguise the English language to protect the African languages, with Jamaican words camouflaging English words allowing the dialect to sound as if it had no English in it, so an English speaker would not be able to understand the Jamaican dialect speaker if that was the latter's intention [9]. In her monograph that describes the lexical inversions that have emerged as a result of the impact of the Rastafari movement in Jamaica, Velma Pollard identifies them as expansions within a creole system that the youth have come to hear not only from the Rastaman but in the music of the airwaves. She also suggests that the language has become separated from the burden of the message and become incorporated into the everyday speech of Jamaican people, reflecting the revolution taking place in the Black Afro-Caribbean diaspora around the world today [10]. Revered Jamaican sociologist, academician, choreographer, and dancer Rex Nettleford noted that the Creole of Jamaica, like that of plantation America, represents an authentic expression of organic revolt. He saw it as an appropriate if anguished response to some of the deepest social forces which have shaped and still determine the dynamics of Caribbean society [11]. He quotes Theodor Adorno in putting this revolution in perspective: 'Social protest manifests itself in language change. For defiance of society includes defiance of its language' [12]. Nettleford was a member of a team from the University of the West Indies who authored a pioneering *Report on the Rastafari Movement in Kingston, Jamaica* [13] in 1960 that helped to shape a growing understanding of this profound evolving movement that has catalyzed a growing renaissance of Black people worldwide. One of the leaders of the movement in the 1970s was Mortimo 'Kumi' Planno, himself a great Rasta drummer and 'elder', who was very supportive of the revolutionary changes being made at Bellevue Hospital. Planno led a delegation of elder Rastafari dreads to visit me at Bellevue in 1979. Bellevue Hospital's *Madnificent Irations* had a profound impact on the Rastafari movement and Jamaican society, as it provided an explication of the movement to people both in Jamaica and in the wider world, in a dramatic form that was cogent and lucid for all races and classes. This play came at a time when the movement was launching itself on the world and having a profound impact in the Caribbean, Africa, Europe, North America, and Australasia. Many of the philosophical and political changes in Bellevue were taking place in the context of Rastafari—of the experiences of Rasta and the political system. From the 1930s onwards Rastafarians indulging in ganja smoking and wearing dreadlocks were called 'mad', arrested by the police for 'madness' and ended up in the mental hospital where their dreadlocks were shaved. They were also forcibly sedated with powerful injectable neuroleptic medications. At Bellevue, we were confronting the entrenched colonial engineering components of madness with the antithesis of that perception of madness. The emerging postcolonial vision of Rasta was that theirs was the sane vision and that the colonial vision was the original madness.

The sociodrama *Madnificent Irations* launched at Bellevue in 1978 clarified this ideological inversion and presented the players of the drama as Rastafari brethren who were tracing their history, which saw Rastafari vilified by British colonialism ending up incarcerated in the colonial madhouse or in prison. The pageant outlined the Rastafari doctrine and philosophy which recognizes Emperor Haile Selassie of Ethiopia as the direct descendant of the Lion of Judah, declaring knowledge of the Emperor as the Almighty, the Conquering Lion of the Tribe of Judah, King of Kings, Lord of Lords, the Alpha and Omega, JAH Rastafari. The symbols and lifestyle including the wearing of dreadlock hairstyles, and the sacramental use of marijuana, have been adopted by Caribbean communities worldwide and were portrayed and predicted in the drama. *Madnificent Irations* challenged the strongly held belief outlined by Ray Prince [14] that the Rastafari movement was involved in criminal and violent anti-establishment activity, and that many Black people engaged in the antithetical transformation to Rastafari were attempting to resolve racial, religious, class, and gender conflicts found in a 'self-racist syndrome' characterized by the negation of their Blackness and the incorporation of Eurocentric concepts of self into their personal identity systems.

In *Madnificent Irations*, Rastafari was portrayed as the cultural manifestation of offspring of a proud tribe of Africans enslaved in the New World engaging to 'beat down Babylon.' 'Babylon'—the name given by the Rastafari movement to the established sociopolitical economic and religious system, which enslaved Africans and brought them to the Americas to work the plantations. Voicing the Biblical prophecy that Babylon must fall and that the Black man will return to Africa from the four corners of the world to which he has been scattered, and demanding an end to exploitation while upholding the Nyabinghi Order, embodying 'death to black and white oppressors' [15], the Rastafari movement has become a powerful revolutionary countercultural force that has swept across the Caribbean and around the world. Made popular internationally by hypnotic reggae music, and reggae superstars, notably Bob Marley, Peter Tosh, and the Third World Band, Rastafari represents a new cultural emergence of the Black man with his own symbols. The spectacular colors of the red, gold, and green of Africa, the use of marijuana in ritual sacrament, and a religious, social, and political philosophy are uniquely central to its existence.

Planno invited the Bellevue players to perform *Madnificent Irations* in the open space behind the Coronation Market at Salt Lane in inner city

Kingston one night, to a huge working-class audience. The importance of putting on this performance in the heart of downtown Kingston, which housed the volatile political constituencies of the two main political parties that were locked in mortal combat at that time in the 1970s, should not be underestimated. Situated just behind the Jamaica Labour Party stronghold of Tivoli Gardens, Coronation Market has been the central axis of trade first for the British as a trading post for slaves, and now as a centre of commerce for the Jamaican people, situated in the heart of the city [16]. Yet this insightful performance, attended by thousands, went almost unnoticed by the rest of Jamaican society.

The message of *Madnificent Irations* also questioned the Babylon orthodoxy of ganja as a cause of madness. In fact, I had gone on a personal medical crusade about the psychological effects of ganja, attacking the conventional widespread medical pronouncements of ganja as a principal cause of psychosis, both at home and abroad. I presented a case study at the prestigious Medical Faculty of the University of the West Indies of a patient who I had successfully treated for alcoholism and personality disorder with ganja; I was a keynote speaker at an international conference on cannabis in Amsterdam in 1980. I had also grown dreadlocks in 1977. The advent of a Senior Medical Officer of Bellevue Hospital being a dreadlocks Rastaman was difficult for Jamaican society to stomach at the time. I had been meeting with Rastafari communities all over the country and providing treatment and care for the brethren who were genuinely mentally ill. *Madnificent Irations* had triggered a sociocultural tsunami that challenged the European colonial concept of madness, had debunked many deep-seated myths about Rastafari, the etiologic role of marijuana in the genesis of madness, and had catalyzed a revolutionary new *community engagement* with the treatment and management of mental illness in Jamaican society. Most importantly, *Madnificent Irations* signaled the launch of psychohistoriographic cultural therapy as a new era in world psychiatry. In his review of my book *Psychohistoriography*, Divine Charura of Leeds Metropolitan University has opined that psychohistoriography is a practical dynamic group process, relevant to all psychotherapeutic work, not just psychoanalysis, and throws light on the cultural issues raised when working with people from minority groups and disadvantaged communities [17]. He has presented psychohistoriography as a formidable challenge to the Western concept of psychoanalysis and its assumed relevance to a non-Western psyche.

Slowly the importance of the work spawned in the bowels of Bellevue Hospital in the late 1970s began gaining traction in Western psychiatry. Some forty years after the launch of this pageant Christina Maechler Williams has described the model of psychohistoriographic cultural therapy developed in the context of Jamaica in the 1970s [18]. She has suggested that it was an answer to existing therapy models that almost exclusively addressed the White middle class of Europe and the USA. In another review of my book, Suman J. Fernando of London Metropolitan University has written that the technique of psychohistoriography and forms of psychotherapy derived from it effectively challenge traditional Western views about the genesis of 'mental illness'. He makes the point that the domination of the non-Western world by the West has had a profound effect on the disciplines of psychology and psychiatry [19]. He describes the process of psychohistoriographic cultural therapy as being particularly useful for professionals in the mental health field working with people from Black and other minority ethnic backgrounds.

There is a view which dismisses the validity of psychotherapy for Black people, and that race plays a crucial role in the psychotherapeutic process. Robert Carter [20] has suggested that some authors, theorists, and researchers have argued that Blacks are not suitable for psychotherapy because of their inherited personality characteristics (e.g., resistance, suspiciousness), their inability to comprehend the nature of psychotherapy (e.g., the verbal self-exploratory process), and the effects of their oppressed status in America and other societies. In addition, he asserts, White middle-class mental health professionals have typically treated Blacks and other visible racial/ethnic group people as if they were devoid of specific cultures. *Madnificent Irations* and psychohistoriographic cultural therapy, which emerged from the creation of this popular theatre pageant, have put paid to such Western psychiatric dogma proclaiming that Black people are devoid of culture, and established a concrete example of a group psychotherapeutic process with demonstrable tangible outcomes for Black people.

When *Madnificent Irations* was created, the technical resources to videotape the process and the pageant were not available. However, the performance text (see Appendix) has been preserved and many photographs were taken that prove irrevocably the existence of this people's revolution. Some of the photographs and newspaper articles written about the performances and the process are presented here to detail the events that surrounded the pageant's creation, and provide a historical benchmark for the experience and its progression, the aftermath of the events and their consequences. In a later chapter I also demonstrate the ease with which politics can destroy physical structures, but that ideas and events emerging from the consciousness of a people cannot easily be eradicated.

The *Gleaner* news item reported on the first performance of *Madnificent Irations*, depicting the history and struggles of the mental hospital in Jamaica, which opened at the institution's Garden Theatre to a packed house on Thursday evening, August 30, 1978. The *Gleaner* article sounded like the review of a sophisticated and established theatrical critic at a conventional Jamaican performance centre. It described the pageantry of historical happenings at the Bellevue Hospital to a large crowd headed by the Governor-General, Florizel Glasspole, Mrs. Michael Manley, the wife of the Prime Minister, and the Parliamentary Secretary in the Ministry of Health, Dr. Winston Davidson. It described the performance as an entertaining blend of song, dance, drama, color, and comedy, which opened with the popular song 'Rivers of Babylon', followed by a short piece, 'Madness the fear', in which a patient tells what it is like to be mad. A folk song, 'Dumariah Mama', was then sung, accompanied by Kumina dancing and congo drumming, with the performers wearing colorful headwraps and dresses. The scenes had titles such as 'Slavery and Emancipation', 'Misinterpreting Culture', 'Rebellion Days', 'The Working Class Wakes Up', and 'Bedward'. Well-known spirituals, accompanied by dancing, kept the audience entertained. They included 'Bright Angels Gather Round,' 'John Saw Them Coming,' 'Roll Jordan Roll,' and 'When My Pilot Come,' and folk songs such as 'Sly Mongoose,' 'Jane and Louisa,' and 'Dip dem Bedward.' One of the brief dramatic pieces which drew much applause was in the first scene, in which a 'madwoman' confronted the doctor on his daily rounds with the question 'Ah who yu?' The audience found it extremely funny when she went on to describe the doctor, although four letter curse words were used in the process. The players were members of staff and patients [21].

Over 75 patients and staff took part in its production, with a *dramatis personae* of fifty performers. All of the 'warm up' and creative techniques developed by the process of creating this first pageant became the fundaments of cultural therapy which would be used in the therapeutic process of rehabilitation in the Cultural Therapy Centre in the years to come. The *Daily Gleaner* of Tuesday, 5 September 1978 published photographs of the audience at the performance and the pageant, with the caption as quoted below (Fig. 4.1).

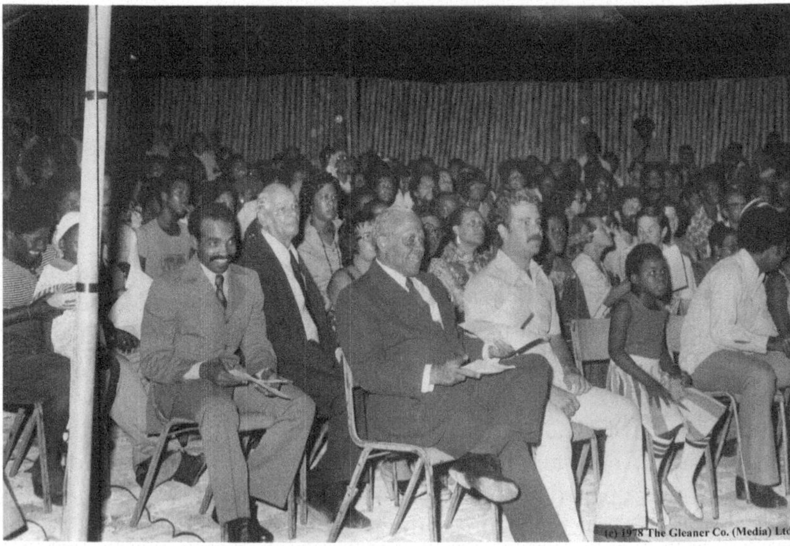

Fig. 4.1 "AT THE PAGEANT: The Governor General, The Most Honorable Florizel Glasspole (Left front row) is amused at some of the antics on stage during a scene from 'Madnificent Irations' which opened at the Garden Theatre, Bellevue Hospital, Kingston on Thursday evening. Behind the Governor General (at left) is his A.D.C. Captain John Prescod". *The Daily Gleaner*, Tuesday, 5 September 1978

Bellevue Hospital has held psychic terror in the hearts and minds of most Jamaican people since its construction in 1862. So to see hundreds of people come out at night to enter the grounds of the mental hospital was indeed a shocking sight. Journalist Cynthia Wilmot reminded us in an article, titled 'A Jamaican Approach to Mental Illness,' in the *Sunday Sun* of the fearsome reputation of the hospital [22]. She described the daily battle to improve conditions, staff members being encouraged by the knowledge of how far they had come from the 'bad old days', when the only form of treatment for madness was restraint, and when patients were treated more like animals than human beings. Wilmot described the early history of the asylum from the first days after its construction in 1861 as a horror story, with tales of madmen lashed to the masts of sailing ships for the tortuous voyage from Montego Bay, and of deranged persons walking halfway across the island, hands manacled, accompanied by a policeman on horseback. She related that once at the asylum, patients were cast into small dungeon-like cells where the only sanitation was provided by a crude hole in the floor, where heavily barred doors clanged shut at sundown to remain locked until morning. These dungeons, she reported, were now happily condemned, for all to see as a grim reminder of the past. Before the establishment of the asylum, she reported, the mentally ill were tucked away shamefully, with only White people being lucky enough to enter it, as mentally ill slaves were imprisoned in cell-like 'hothouses' where, usually, they languished and died. In 1843 the asylum building occupied the site that currently houses the outpatients clinic at Kingston Public Hospital. At that time, chains, leg irons, and stocks were used as restraints, and in some years, more than half of those admitted died. Wilmot wrote that even in those early days there were some physicians who envisioned a new approach to madness. One such was Dr. Alexander Campbell, who scandalized conservative colleagues at the asylum by abolishing the leg irons and chains. Unfortunately, his campaign was cut short by early retirement and the improvements he introduced were short-lived.

Cynthia Wilmot was born in Stratford, Ontario, Canada, in 1921, and met Jamaican Fred Wilmot, a soldier and well-known poet in Toronto; they married in 1942. They moved to Vancouver and worked as reporters for a while, then moved to Winnipeg, where Fred became the first Black editor of a daily newspaper while Cynthia got a reporting job on a Jewish newspaper. They moved to Jamaica in 1951. Her article, 'A Jamaican Approach to Mental Illness' [22], provided an important commentary on the therapeutic revolution that was taking place in Bellevue Hospital and more widely in Jamaica that had begun in the 1960s and 1970s. As a White Canadian domiciled in Jamaica for most of her life [23], she was in an excellent position to interpret the changes that were taking place in the country, and in mental health specifically. Much of the history reported in her article was previously captured in the sociodrama activities of the 1970s. The launch of *Madnificent Irations* in the bowels of Bellevue Hospital in August 1978 represented an *in vivo* attempt to trace the development of psychiatric social systems and therapeutic models that have evolved in Jamaica to counter the ideology of violent insanity that has developed *pari passu* with the development of capitalism, enslavement, and colonial exploitation. The pageant portrayed five significant periods in Caribbean history: pre-colonial; slavery; post-emancipation; later colonial; and post-independence. The discussions that emerged at the ethnohistorical meetings in Bellevue Hospital in early 1978 posited that the imposed philosophy of the colonizer created an ideology of psychopathology in the colonized and an institutional framework of involuntary commitment and custodialization. The pageant attempted to describe the parallel symbiosis of Western psychiatry and traditional medicine in Jamaica in the context of European colonization of this region and the metamorphosis toward holistic mental health that has reinforced traditional healing models and negated involuntary commitment and coercive treatment through community engagement and recovery. The pageant suggested that the psychiatric ideologies and institutions arising from the colonizer culture have been systematically confronted and resisted by an emerging politically independent Jamaica, and that the diagnostic and psychopathological constructions of the colonizer are being replaced by the emerging mental health creations of the newly liberated Jamaican people. Most importantly, the pageant reminded us that the Jamaica in which the Lunatic Asylum was conceived and built was dominated and controlled by White Britishers and their offspring White Jamaicans; that the British were brutish and that there was a deep and distinct schism between the Whites who were powerful and wealthy, and the Blacks who were poor and owned little, with little social power. The only function of the Black underclass was to provide service for the Whites who ruled. The pageant reminded us of the social and historical origin of the world of the 'haves' and the 'have nots' and the coterminous relationship between race and class.

Bibliography

1. Hickling FW (1985) Poem "Westminster System" (Unpublished).
2. Hickling FW, Robertson-Hickling H (2007) Cultural Therapy and Reasonable Accommodation. Presentation and workshop at The Division of Social and Cultural Psychiatry, McGill University, and The Centre for the Arts in Human Development, Concordia University. https://www.mcgill.ca/tcpsych/files/tcpsych/Psychohistoriography.pdf.
3. Hickling FW (1989) Sociodrama in the Rehabilitation of Chronic Mental Illness. *Hospital and Community Psychiatry, 40*, 402–406.
4. Neologism (n.d.) From Wikipedia, the free encyclopaedia. http://en.wikipedia.org/wiki/Neologism.
5. Berrios GE (2009) Neologisms. *History of Psychiatry, 20*, 480–496.
6. Jaspers K (1913) *General Psychopathology*. Translated from the German by J Hoenig and MW Hamilton (1963). Manchester, UK: Manchester University Press.

7. Magnificent (n.d.) http://www.thesaurus.com/browse/magnificent.
8. Bennett L (1993) *Auntie Roachy Seh.* ed. M Morris. Kingston: Sangster's Book Stores Ltd., p. 1.
9. Morris M (1993) *Introduction* from Louise Bennett, *Auntie Roachy Seh.* ed. Mervyn Morris. Kingston: Sangster's Book Stores Ltd., p. vii.
10. Pollard V (1994) *Dread Talk: The Language of Rastafari.* London: Taylor & Francis, pp. 49–56.
11. Nettleford RM (1978) *Caribbean Cultural Identity: The Case of Jamaica.* Kingston: Institute of Jamaica, pp. 187, 189.
12. Nettleford RM (1978) *Caribbean Cultural Identity: The Case of Jamaica.* Kingston: Institute of Jamaica, p. 18, note 29.
13. Smith MG, Augier R, Nettleford R (1960) *Report on the Rastafari Movement in Kingston, Jamaica.* Kingston: Institute of Social and Economic Research, University of the West Indies, Mona.
14. Prince R (1969) The Rastafari of Jamaica: A Study of Group Beliefs and Social Stress. Presented at a meeting of the American Psychiatric Association—Caribbean Psychiatric Association, Ocho Rios, Jamaica, *Transcultural Psychiatric Research Review,* 7(1), 58–62.
15. Philos F (1935) Secret Society to Destroy Whites. *The Jamaica Times,* December 7.
16. *The Gleaner* (2012) Destination Downtown; The Birthplace of Jamaican Music; The Centre of Business and Commerce. http://www.digjamaica.com/destinationdowntown.
17. Charura D (2012) Psychohistoriography: A Post-colonial Psychoanalytic and Psychotherapeutic Model by Frederick W Hickling. Book Reviews. *Therapy Today, 24*(7), 46.
18. Williams CM (2014) *Psychohistoriographic Cultural Therapy,* MSc thesis, Department of Psychotherapy and Biopsychosocial Health at Danube University Krems, Winterthur, Austria.
19. Fernando SJ (2013) Book Review: Psychohistoriography: A Post-Colonial Psychoanalytic and Psychotherapeutic Model. *British Journal of Psychiatry, 203,* 77.
20. Carter RT (1995) *The Influence of Race and Racial Identity in Psychotherapy: Toward a Racially Inclusive Model.* Chichester: Wiley.
21. *The Daily Gleaner* (1978) Full House Sees Opening of 'Madnificent Irations', September 5.
22. Wilmot C (1980) A Jamaican Approach to Mental Illness, *Sunday Sun,* December 28.
23. Reckord M (2003) Cynthia Wilmot—A Lifetime of Writing and Film Making. *Jamaica Gleaner,* Sunday, June 8.

CHAPTER 5

Mobilizing Bellevue by Building the Garden Theatre

So how are we to expect
a system which protects
The rights of private property
To treat Black man with respect? [1]

The process of cultural therapy emerged in Jamaica in the 1970s in the context of the rapidly changing ideological climate shortly after the attainment of political independence from Great Britain. Struggling with the psychiatric imperatives of community psychiatry and deinstitutionalization and the need to find a therapeutic vehicle which would unite widely diverse outlooks and expectations of patients and workers who were at different professional, educational, ideological and class levels, the aim was to bring about therapeutic change, the mobilization of production, to facilitate destigmatization, and to promote mental health education in the community. A major element of the transformation of the mental hospital, and its conversion from a custodial into a rehabilitative hospital was the development of the cultural therapy process and the formation of the Cultural Therapy Centre at Bellevue Hospital. Cultural therapy was pioneered in 1977.

The therapeutic community, together with an open door policy, was instituted at Bellevue in 1973, initially as a pilot rehabilitation unit of 50 beds; it was then extended throughout the hospital [2]. In the 1970s, therapeutic community group meetings were established on all 24 wards and were held daily between patients and staff. Vocational and cultural

F. W. Hickling, *Decolonization of Psychiatry in Jamaica*,
https://doi.org/10.1007/978-3-030-48489-7_5

therapy programs offering arts, drama, dance, and music therapy were offered to all patients in the hospital [3]. The therapeutic community policy achieved a significant positive beneficial impact on the outcome of patient care as well as on the attitudes of staff and patients to psychiatric care. All long-stay patients were moved into designated rehabilitation wards graded by clinical assessment, assessed risk, vocational ability, and community family contact. Vocational areas and activities were created in the institution to provide constructive occupation for the patients. The nursing administration then agreed to move one member of staff from each of the 24 custodial wards of the hospital into the newly created Bellevue Cultural Therapy Centre to initiate their new rehabilitative roles. Before starting their functions in this new area, these staff members were sent on a 14-week course of training at the Edna Manley College of the Visual and Performing Arts (EMCVPA). This Centre was an amalgam of four schools of art, drama, music, and dance.

My early experience in the Jamaican cultural scene significantly influenced the development of the cultural therapy movement. Apart from being a psychiatrist in Jamaica for nearly 50 years, I have been involved in entertainment and theatre productions for an even longer period. On leaving Wolmer's High School for Boys, having been active in the school's drama club, I started working with performers with the Jamaica Festival Movement in the early 1960s, such as the Skatalites Band, Hortense Ellis, Toots and the Maytals, and many others. I was the stage manager for the National Dance Theatre Company (NDTC) for 15 years during which time I gained significant expertise at home and abroad in the production and management of stage performances.

I had just turned sixteen when I was invited to help with the stage management of the newly formed NDTC. I had been working at the time as a clerk at the offices of the Jamaica Independence Celebrations Committee, an organization which had been set up to plan the festivities for the upcoming celebration of independence from British colonial rule. One of the Committee members was Jamaican Rhodes scholar and University of the West Indies professor Rex Nettleford, who was the other co-founder and artistic director of the NDTC. I joined Felix Barnett to become one of the first stage managers of the NDTC, a job that I held for 15 years, and which would fundamentally influence my life.

Rex Nettleford certainly has been one of Jamaica's most successful sons. Born in Montego Bay in extremely poor circumstances, Rex's superior intellect and talent propelled him first through the fledgling University of the West Indies (UWI) as one of its first pupils, and then as a Rhodes Scholar at Oxford University. On his return to Jamaica in the late 1950s, he went into leadership overdrive first as a director of the Trade Union Education Institute and lecturer at UWI. He also pioneered the NDTC. A strikingly handsome Black man with formidable intellectual and artistic skills and talent, Rex was to influence my development profoundly. He represented the generation of Jamaicans who were striding resolutely into the uncharted seas of postcolonialism and embodied the epitome of the emerging African-Jamaican intellectual and leader, performing a multifaceted role in a number of different arenas. He was later to become the Vice Chancellor of UWI and was selected as one of four honorary doctorates at Oxford University in 2003, to commemorate the centenary of the Rhodes Scholarship. He was a prolific writer, a challenging teacher and a superbly talented dancer, choreographer, and academic scholar. As stage manager of the NDTC, I had to work very closely with him in the execution of the overall running of the dance theatre performance, and soon became a pupil of this hard-driving mentor. Ambitious and demanding, Rex drove himself and those who worked with him mercilessly. I learned very early that if one wanted to find him during the course of any day, the best chances of success would be to go to his office at six in the morning. Invariably, he would be found pounding away at his typewriter, hours before his staff came to work. He told me that he had acquired that habit early in life and would confound his fellow students at university by typing all his lectures and assignments almost immediately after they were given. Rex was the most skillful and fluent two-finger typist that I have ever come across. As I sit here two-finger typing at six in the morning, I give thanks for his mentorship.

Rex's talent was blinding and his leadership formidable. I learned at first hand the connection between artistic creativity and its political and philosophical grounding. I watched him preparing himself and other dancers by rigorous repetitive training exercises, skillful, and bold artistic creation, which challenged orthodoxy, and then the distillation of these creative products into profound philosophical essays that hammered out the elements of culture as a political and transformatory weapon. He was also extremely articulate and a skillful manipulator of the English language, skills which I have keenly attempted to emulate. I will never forget an experience in London in 1965 when the NDTC was on tour in England as part of the Commonwealth Festival of Arts, when Rex was asked to give an *extempore* presentation to a large group of international journalists at South Africa House. His speech was formidable in intellectual content, artistic and academic profundity, language control, and articulateness. Here was a Black man, a descendant of an African enslaved in the New World, who epitomized the social engineering of colonialism and slavery, who was teaching the English how to speak, how to think, and how to be creative, *in their own language*! Also, this was a time when White supremacists were staging an all-out last stand to maintain White supremacist hegemony in Ian Smith's Rhodesia, and in apartheid South Africa.

A major development of the 1970s in Jamaica was the incorporation of all the schools of the cultural arts into the EMCVPA. Spearheaded by the Institute of Jamaica and by stalwarts such as Rex Nettleford (dance), Jerry Craig (art) and Pamela O'Gorman (music) [4], they fused the School of Arts and the Jamaica School of Music with new Schools of Drama and Dance, housed in a modern creative complex in the center of Kingston. Many of my friends and colleagues involved in the theatre and dance had been appointed as lecturers and tutors. As soon as the idea of a Cultural Therapy Centre at Bellevue began to take place, to take root, to take shape, I went to see the Principals from the Schools of Music, Dance and Drama and made arrangements to train 30 psychiatric aides from Bellevue Hospital.

Many members of the NDTC were leading tutors at these schools. Marjorie Whylie, Musical Director of the NDTC, was a Tutor at the School of Music. Sheila Barnett, Barbara Requa, Bert Rose, and Barry Moncrieffe, dancers in the NDTC, were all Tutors at the School of Dance. Dennis Scott and Hortencer Lindsay were leading tutors at the School of Drama. They all played an important role in shaping this training program for the workers of the mental hospital. The local news media recorded the significance of the event. *The Star* of June 30, 1977 [5] reported the development of the training of psychiatric aides at the EMCVPA. Journalist Beverly Hamilton [6] commented on the graduation exercises of this group of Bellevue workers, noting that the use of the arts as a form of therapy would soon materialize in Bellevue Hospital, when 30 psychiatric aides and assistant nurses graduated from a foundation course in the arts and returned to the workplace to put their newly found skills into practice. The Cultural Therapy Unit program represented a blend of three modern psychiatric concepts—rehabilitation, democratization, and the use of the arts in therapy. It was realized that any transformatory move from custodialization toward rehabilitation required involvement of the ancillary workers. For this reason, they were chosen first to receive training about the arts so that they could develop a therapy program for Bellevue patients. They were taught the use of basic choral singing techniques, a range of Jamaican folk songs, and integrated song and dance routines as they were taught the movements of traditional folk dances commonly performed in Kumina and Pocomania ceremonies, as well as dramatic dance improvisations such as the "ball dance" where a bouncing ball was used to counterpoint the rhythm of the music.

The original Cultural Therapy Centre at Bellevue used an essentially conventional psychiatric hospital staffing team structure. Located on the grounds of the hospital, with close access to the adjacent community, it consisted of a clinical support building, attached to a fully equipped open-air garden theatre capable of seating fifteen hundred people, and supported a ten-piece popular musical band. The service welcomed drop-in mentally ill homeless. The majority of participants were residents of the surrounding communities. The therapeutic community principles described by Maxwell Jones in 1968 [7] essentially involved altering the typical social structure of a psychiatric hospital, introducing a community environment that would have a long-lasting, positive effect on the mental condition of patients. In the therapeutic community, the social structure of the ward is characteristically different from that of more traditional hospital ward units. An attempt is made to involve the entire community of staff, patients, and their relatives in treatment and administration. There is emphasis on free communication within and between staff and patient groups and on permissive attitudes that encourage free expression of feelings. These factors imply a democratic, egalitarian community rather than a traditional hierarchical social organization. In a therapeutic community, traditional mental hospital concepts and behaviors are abandoned, and staff and patient roles and role-relationships are the subject of frequent examination and discussion. The aim of this practice is to increase the effectiveness of roles and to sharpen the community's perception of them. This decentralization or democratization of authoritarianism creates an atmosphere which Jones called a *therapeutic culture*, which emphasizes active rehabilitation, permissiveness, and cooperation and attempts to resocialize institutionalized people into the role of active normal human beings once more. The essential feature of the therapeutic community, however, is the reliance on the group dynamic to break down dissension and hostility between staff and patients, and to increase communication and engender resocialization for all concerned.

Our formula for the implementation of this process in Bellevue included daily group meetings in every ward of the hospital and the establishment of the large group ethnohistorical meeting. Based on the African oral tradition of group communication, and led by a nominated chairperson, groups of ten and upward would meet on a daily basis to discuss their histories and activities, employing anecdotes and folk material such as ring games, storytelling, and improvisation [8]. The similarity to the Tavistock Model of group activity in the UK [9] is noted, with the recognition that the activities grew out of the cultural oral tradition activities which had been passed down from the African tradition through slavery rather than the incorporation of a model of intensive learning drawing on the work of British psychoanalysts.

Large Group Ethnohistorical Meetings

Having piloted the therapeutic community and rehabilitation principles in a 40-bed Rehabilitation Unit at Bellevue, I was promoted to the role of Senior Medical Officer (SMO) in 1976. As the chief administrator of the hospital, management of its nearly 2000 workers was a prime assignment in tandem with the clinical management of the 2400 resident patients. The staff were highly politicized and were represented by five of the local trade unions—The Bustamante Industrial Trade Union, the National Workers Union, the Trade Union Council, The Nurses Association and the Jamaica Union of Public Officers and Public Employees. In 1978, Rex Nettleford and Carl Stone, in conjunction with the political directions of the People's National Party (PNP) government, led by Michael Manley, had written a manual on worker participation [10] which had been introduced to the burgeoning trade union movement in Jamaica in a national effort to increase productivity [11]. The period of 1976 was extremely critical for Jamaica. It was during that time that the PNP received an overwhelming plebiscite at the polls to carry out a program of political transformation in Jamaica. Manley's party sold that plebiscite on the rhetoric of *Democratic Socialism*. The politics of the 1970s has been analysed exhaustively by a number of authors, not the least of whom was Manley himself, who wrote several books on the period. The present narrative is about the struggle for the mental health of the Jamaican people and the role the mental hospital played in that process of decolonization.

The country's attention was focused on what form this process of transformation to democratic socialism would take. A Ministry of Mobilization had been set up under the leadership of the General Secretary of the PNP, dental surgeon Dr. D.K. Duncan. One of the objectives of that ministry was to produce a program which would mobilize the productivity of the unemployed and under-employed people of Jamaica, and to transform the social productivity modes of this bastion of British colonialism in the Caribbean. The vehicle of transformation of the productive modes of society was the mechanism of worker participation, and, as mentioned above, an authoritative book was published by two eminent professors at UWI, Carl Stone and Rex Nettleford. My intention was to combine this concept of worker participation with my own psychotherapeutic insights to create the vehicle of transformation and decolonization of the mental hospital. The participation of man in running the affairs of his life, his work, and his environment has been the thrust of the politics of freedom and the ideology of empowerment worldwide for centuries. The possible models of economic participatory systems exist on a spectrum of alternatives ranging from state, social, or socialist ownership, to private ownership. The models distinguish clearly between self-management based on economic self-determination and capital-controlled or dehumanized systems as polar opposites on this spectrum. Stone and Nettleford highlighted the legacy of deprivation and powerlessness of Jamaican workers and identified authoritarianism in management practices in the workplace as a direct result of the Jamaican slave plantation experience, now reflected in deeply entrenched class distinctions (Fig. 5.1). It was in this context that a worker participation program was implemented at Bellevue in 1977.

The Bellevue adaptation of the 'Town Hall' meeting concept was one of our practical interpretations of the worker participation principles, which we called *ethnohistorical meetings* (Fig. 5.2).

As a result there was much hostility, resentment and worker frustration, symptomatic of the state of chronic institutionalization of the hospital. It is in this context that the concept of sociodrama was conceived, as a method of quickly and easily creating a historical understanding of the process of psychiatry in Jamaica. At one of these meetings, we decided collectively that the workers at Bellevue would create a pageant

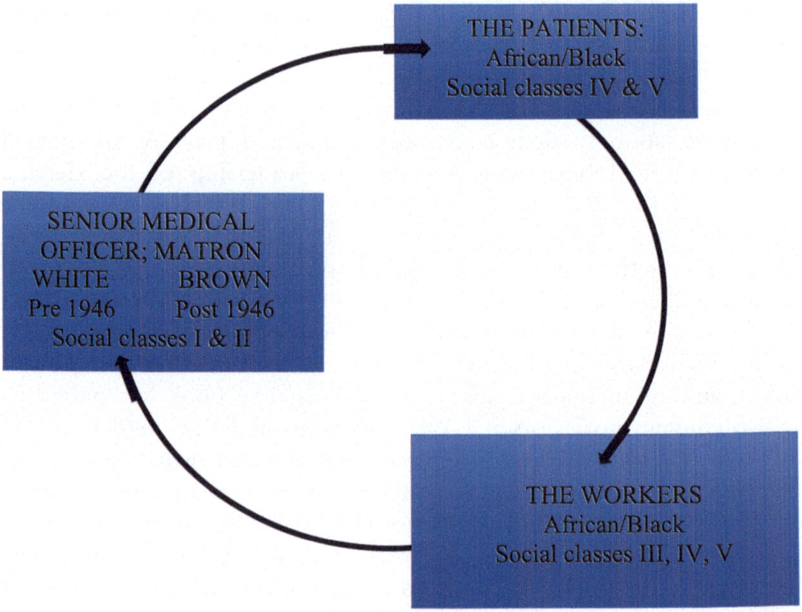

Fig. 5.1 The racial/class dialectic

depicting the history of the institution from the perspective of the people who lived and worked within the institution, relying on the skills and talents of a core team of 30 assistant nurses and psychiatric aides who had been trained the previous year at the EMCVPA. The objectives of the sociodrama were to shatter the myths surrounding mental illness, to rehabilitate the mentally ill, to raise the social and political consciousness of patients and workers, to mobilize productivity within the institution, and to use the culture of the people as a natural catalyst of development.

The ethnohistorical meetings involved a special meeting of workers and patients, where 15 of the oldest persons from the hospital were selected as historical discussants. The persons were workers and patients who had been within the institution for longer than 40 years. It was their job to free associate on their memories of the institution, of clinical practices, anecdotes, political happenings from their own experiences and from their own historical knowledge.

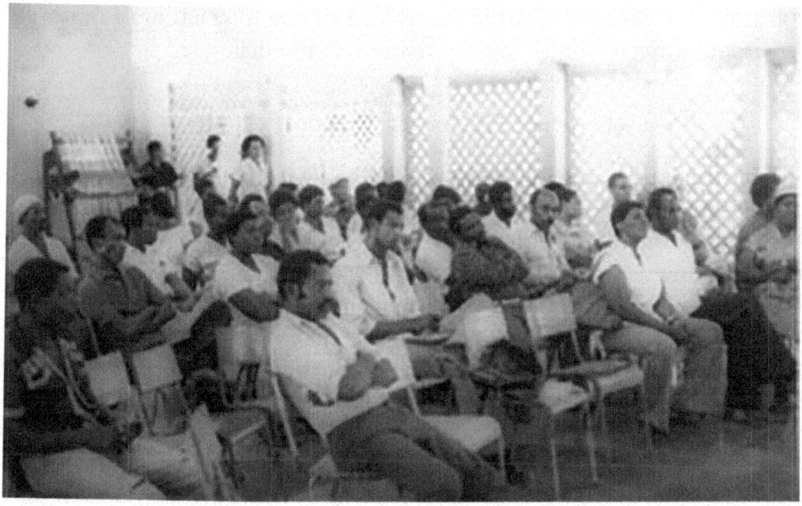

Fig. 5.2 Patients, nurses, and other staff members participating in a large group ethnohistorical meeting, 1978

This free association of historical perception by the oldest historians was then discussed critically by the other workers and patients present, and differences of opinion and opposing perceptions of historical events were aired. The meetings discussed the historical facts which emerged in the context of the political climate of Jamaica and the wider international perspectives. The meetings were tape-recorded, and as might have been expected, the dynamics produced surprises, contradictions, arguments, and conflicts, and acted as a collective historical catharsis. The meetings tried to establish chronological historical frameworks for introspection and self-examination, to understand the cultural and political perspectives from matron to hospital aide, from SMO to sanitation worker, from chief cook to supply clerk and from secretary to occupational therapist. From this, different dialectical perspectives emerged.

The main themes soon became clear. The most striking was the perception of the patients as being oppressed, as victims of an oppressive socio-political and economic system, set up within the racist context of British colonialization, where workers were treated only a little better than the patients. These realizations were now being made clear to the collective consciousness of the institution by the interaction of opposing forces and ideas within the group reasoning and dialogue.

The Madness/Badness Violence Dialectic

Stigma, madness and behavior were also argued out at the ethnohistorical meeting as being a social perception of abnormal behavior. This discussion came in the context of the murder of a male patient by another patient on 'B' Ward that had occurred some days before. This was identified by the meeting participants as 'Murder as Madness'. It was located in what the meeting saw as the 'Mirror of Murder', where the death row murderers who had participated in the breakout at the St. Catherine District Prison [12] in 1976 were being identified as 'Murder as Badness', in dialectical opposition to the Jamaican guerrillas who fought with guns and politics, who were seen by the British colonial authorities as being 'bad' (Fig. 5.3). Both 'Murder as Madness' and 'Murder as Badness' were located within the dialectical continuum of the 'Mirror of Murder' and thus related to the 'Murder of War', as reflected in the politically motivated Green Bay Massacre, a covert operation carried out by special forces in the Jamaica Defence Force (JDF) on January 5, 1978, one of the darkest and most controversial days in Jamaica's history [13]. With the promise of guns and jobs in the military if they co-operated with the government, 14 men were lured into an ambush at the Green Bay Firing Range in St. Catherine, allegedly by members of the Military Intelligence Unit. Five of the men were killed, and the remainder fled to nearby bushes. At least one entered the bay and was rescued by a passing fishing boat. The men were all from the Jamaica Labour Party (JLP) stronghold of Southside in central Kingston. An official report from the JDF said that the men who died were shot dead after they were surprised by soldiers doing target practice at the JDF firing range.

It was clear to us that this behavior on the part of the individuals concerned resulted from the contradictions of a sick socioeconomic political system. It was also clear that the ruling classes had created the madhouse to deter people who were promoting cultural and political ideas that were antithetical to the ruling culture. Finally, we could see that the prison had been conceived and built along similar architectural lines to those of its twin sister, constructed around the same time—the Jamaica Lunatic Asylum. The insights emerging from the ethnohistoriographic

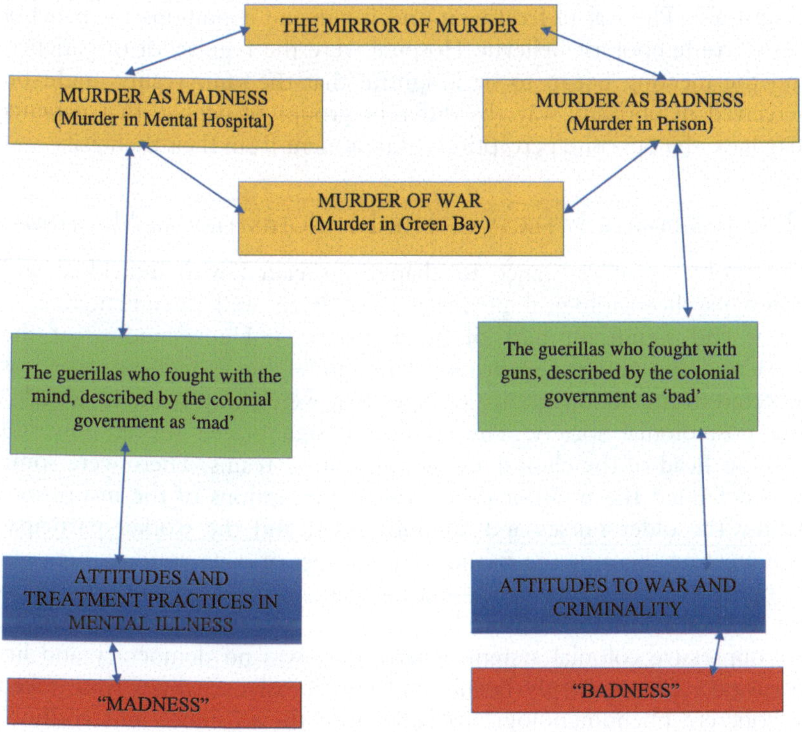

Fig. 5.3 The madness/badness violence dialectic

meetings were startling to all, especially when we began to examine the perception of history that represented the 'moral treatment' system of Dr. Thomas Allen in 1863 as moral and humane. The collective memory of the situation was just the opposite, with custodialization, enforced labor and later electroconvulsive therapy, intravenous sedation and locked rooms as the concrete perception of the oppression. The 1873 Lunatic Asylum Law crafted by Allen made the mentally ill into criminals by fixing in law the reality that for persons with psychoses to obtain treatment, they first had to be seen by a Resident Magistrate and a Justice of the Peace before being 'sentenced' to the Lunatic Asylum. The police had the right to arrest any person they found 'wandering at large' or 'behaving in an abnormal manner' and bring them before a

Magistrate. Physical ill-treatment and inhumane conditions for patients in the contemporary Bellevue Hospital were the regular lot of patients, and the meeting began to be insightful that the same reality might be perceived in opposite ways by different groups of people, that patients may have the opposite perceptions of treatment from their therapists.

The Immediate Effects of the Ethnohistorical Meetings

The problems of resistance to change associated with individual and group psychosociological processes have been well documented as a major and significant part of these processes. Understanding of the impact of the colonial institutional design of the mental hospital was reflected in the administrative changes that were being made by a fledgling postcolonial society. The colonial design placed the all-powerful SMO as head of the clinical and administrative teams. There were some who defended the traditional benevolent perceptions of the institution, mainly the older nurses and administrators, and the worker participation meetings became the forum for a number of open conflicts between themselves, on the one hand, and ancillary workers on the other who accused these nurses and administrators of being the actual agents of the oppressive colonial system, where there was no democracy and little justice. These sharply hostile and conflictual exchanges were taken as concrete phenomenological examples of the existence and continuation of the class struggle between various groups of workers; this was to manifest in real worker struggle, as subsequently demonstrated. This realization was as startling as the verbalizations which indicated that the workers were just as afraid of the patients as any layman, and that in some unexplained way the total institution was the actual instigator and perpetrator of the societal stigma attaching to madness.

Almost immediately a period of intense industrial unrest emerged spontaneously when the nursing administration attempted to lay off some temporary ancillary workers, who went on strike to protest the decision. At the subsequent arbitration meeting the SMO sided with the ancillary workers. The strike that exploded shut down the hospital for 24 hours, requiring intervention from the police, trade union leaders and officials from the Ministry of Health. The strike caused chaos, with the hospital requiring the military being called on to provide food and security for the patients in the 24 hospital wards. In a counterstrike, a group of 120 registered nurses mounted their own industrial protest.

This period of hot-tempered worker confrontation took place only a few days after the ethnohistorical meeting that had aired the seething hostility between the various classes of workers, which had emerged as verbal clashes between ancillary workers and nursing administration and patients and nurses. It was as if a festering abscess had been lanced! The next three years provided the situation and the wherewithal whereby many of the rigid institutionalized clinical and administrative practices inherited from 100 years of colonial custodial practices were confronted, worked through, and resolved.

In the case of the therapeutic transformation of Bellevue Hospital, the process of resistance was exposed by this trade union dispute by the nursing staff. With the new move to convert Bellevue from a custodial institution into a therapeutic community, the major areas of resistance came from the senior nurses of the nursing administration. Following the dangerous period of worker unrest the group of registered nurses petitioned the government, demanding my removal as SMO of Bellevue Hospital. The nurses alleged that the actions of the SMO, combined with industrial action, had had 'a disastrous effect on patient care and staff morale… and that the interest of the hospital would be better served by his immediate removal…' The matter was taken to a Commission of Enquiry chaired by Attorney at Law David Muirhead QC. The Commission was held at Headquarters House, the building which in the previous century had housed the Legislative Council of the British Colonial Government of Jamaica. The Commission of Enquiry was careful and methodical and lasted for several weeks. The Muirhead Commission interviewed dozens of people of all walks of life within and without Bellevue Hospital. All factions were represented by their legal counsel. The Commission finally ruled that the therapeutic community change processes being implemented at the hospital were legal and appropriate, and the striking nurses were reprimanded and ordered back to work. The Commission reported that the SMO had behaved in an appropriate manner, was exonerated of the charges laid against him by the nursing staff, and the demands of the registered nurses were rejected. However, the SMO was reprimanded for the use of indecent language to the matron of the mental hospital.

By the end of 1977, the worker participation/therapeutic transformation program was in full swing, and Bellevue Hospital was flourishing. We had established a callaloo farm (callaloo is a vegetable resembling spinach) on three acres of land, and we were now beginning to supply a significant proportion of the local market's demand for it in Kingston. Twice weekly, vendors from the Coronation Market would come to the hospital to purchase this vegetable (some smart alec had dubbed them 'crazy greens'). We had established a chicken farm in the area which used to house the criminal lunatics, and we were now producing 1000 chickens per week, which we sold to our kitchen for our own domestic needs. Large group meetings were now being held on every ward on a daily basis, and most of the patients in the hospital were spending the entire day outside of their ward areas in one vocational area or another. The clinical care of the patients had improved tremendously, and now there were almost daily teaching sessions around the hospital which were being attended by nursing students from the different nursing schools in Kingston, and by medical students from UWI. The transformation of Bellevue was occurring, and the government's worker participation program was working. Wildcat strikes, which had been running at 20 per year, had now stopped altogether.

During the period following the eventful ethnohistorical meeting, the group of registered nurses boycotted the development of the cultural therapy activities and refused to participate in the creation of *Madnificent Irations*. To these nurses, the sociodrama process represented a negative, destructive process, and they voiced and acted out their opinions. Following the Muirhead inquiry, the nursing administrators acknowledged the errors of their ways and quickly moved to fill the leadership and administrative vacuum in the burgeoning hospital cultural therapy movement, which they had shunned. They assigned a fully trained nursing sister to run the cultural therapy movement and directed registered nurses to work in conjunction with the assistant nurses and psychiatric aides who had completely taken over the running of these programs without registered nurse supervision. This forced the resistance of the registered nurses underground, only to re-emerge through the national political processes that were heralded by the change of government in Jamaica following the general election in 1980.

Journalist Horace Levy, commenting on the conflict at Bellevue, reported that a number of nurses partially suspended their services and were threatening strike action in support of their demand for an inquiry by the Ministry of Health into the administrative behavior of the SMO (i.e. me) [14]. He reported that the central complaint was that the SMO encouraged auxiliary staff to be disrespectful to nurses and to supervisory staff, thereby encouraging indiscipline. Levy described Bellevue as having been operated for generations under the custodial system of keeping patients confined to their wards and quarters. The idea was to keep them quiet, locked away. Levy mentioned that it was unfortunate that the route by which nurses obtain advancement carries them into administration, where they lose direct contact with patient care. Many of these administrative tasks could be carried out by less specialized clerical staff. The area offering the greatest challenge to nurses and the most crucial of the therapeutic activities has been that of the therapeutic community.

The Cultural Therapy Centre

The program had no performing space in which to carry out our activities. In the initial period, we had to share the facilities in the Occupational Therapy Centre. The challenge was creating a performing centre with little or no money. Most theatres in Jamaica had developed in the context of limited resources. I had watched and assisted in the growth and development of different theatre facilities in Jamaica in my adolescent years. I watched the growth of the Little Theatre not far from my home in Kingston as a teenager, and virtually lived on the building site of the Philip Sherlock Centre for the Creative Arts at UWI in the mid-1960s. I had performed in theatres around the world, and as a stage manager I had extensive knowledge and experience of building sets and scenery and installing electrical lighting and musical sound equipment. The absence of a dedicated performance space at Bellevue was, to me, not an obstacle, but an exciting challenge.

The most suitable location, beside the cultural therapy office, was identified. We chose this site in the northwestern corner of the hospital grounds, a beautiful grove studded with naturally existing lignum vitae and tamarind trees situated between the Cultural Therapy Centre and the playing field. The beautiful purple flower of the lignum vitae tree is the national flower of Jamaica; together with the unique dark green leaves of the hardwood tree, it provided a perfect background for the proposed Garden Theatre. It was not hard to convince Jamaican architect Pat Staniger at the Jamaican government-owned Urban Development Corporation to collaborate on the project, and Pat soon produced a novel concept of circles within circles, creating plans and drawings for the stunningly beautiful Cultural Therapy Centre. The concept of the circle within and without the circle incorporated all of the beautiful trees into its design (Fig. 5.4).

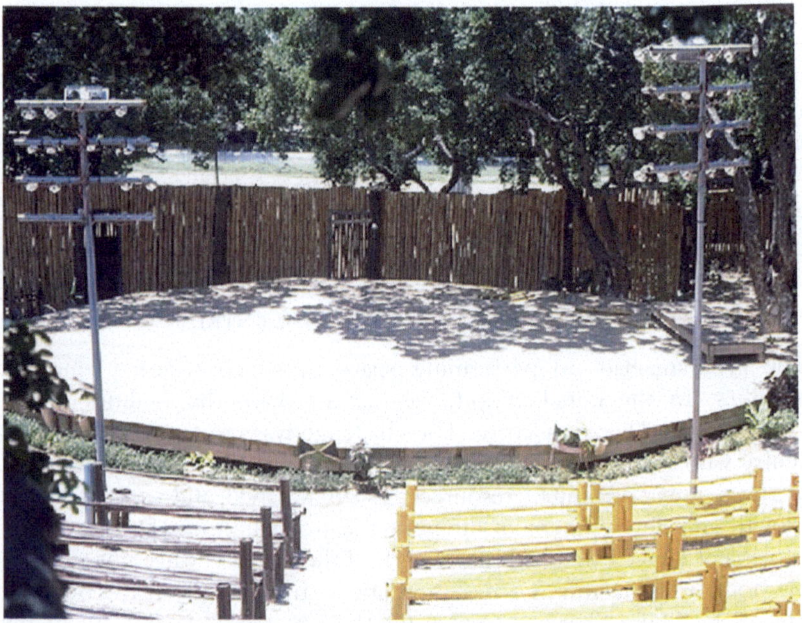

Fig. 5.4 Bellevue Garden Theatre, 1978. The concept of the circle within a circle: a circular stage of bamboo and wood surrounded by a circle of lignum vitae trees

The Jamaican theatre experience was built on the concept of contributions from the community [15]. There had never been budgets or stipends for cultural development in our country. Theatrical groups and in particular stage managers of these groups had become adept at soliciting contributions for theatrical ventures from private and public organizations and individuals.

The stage was based on the concept of the 'theatre in the round' and was a huge circle within the circle of the open-air auditorium. We set to the task of building the theatre without money! By identifying key benefactors (taking care to emphasise the plight of the mental hospital and the mentally ill) and by also soliciting support from the general public, we were able to persuade the Jamaican people to contribute generously to the project. The Jamaica Public Service (the local electricity company) donated two dozen (slightly damaged) wooden electrical poles that we used to provide the foundation for the structure. A local hardware company donated treated pine lumber to build the stage. Abdulla (Johnny) Marzouca, owner of the biggest private lighting company in Jamaica, donated all the electrical wire conduits and outdoor lighting for the facility. The Jamaican Army's engineering division provided, free of charge, earthmoving equipment and operators to prepare the site and grade the slope of the auditorium. Then we set about building it ourselves. Mr. Green, one of the hospital's carpenters, became our foreman and technical adviser. There was no shortage of physical labor, male and female, to carry out the thousand and one tasks required to build this simple but elegant design.

Workers and patients from all over the hospital volunteered their labor. The hospital kitchen sent the patients' meals to the worksite instead of to their wards to facilitate the process. Teams of workers and patients made numerous journeys into the countryside to cut down bamboo, which grows in profusion all over the island. The bamboo became the walls and the seats of the Garden Theatre (Fig. 5.5). The Theatre

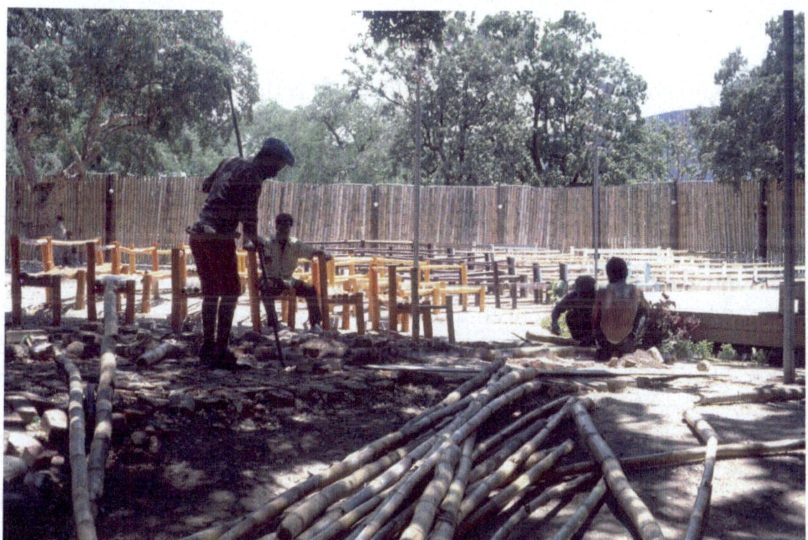

Fig. 5.5 Hospital workers and patients preparing bamboo poles prior to building the exterior wall. Bamboo became a motif of the theatre

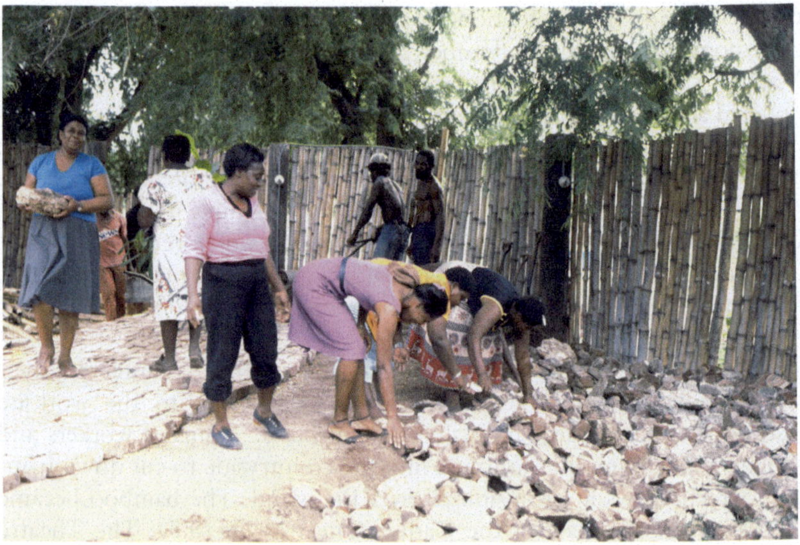

Fig. 5.6 Workers and patients, both male and female, laying the bricks to make the floor

became known euphemistically as the 'bamboo theatre.' Red bricks from an abandoned ward in the institution were recycled to form the floor of the theatre. They had been shipped from England and used to build the asylum in the nineteenth century. They were used as ballast for the ships, which sailed without cargo on the outward voyage from England, but returned laden with the produce of the colonial plantations, primarily sugar and bananas. We felt that this was a fitting resting place for these bricks, which had experienced a century of exploitation and oppression. If those bricks could talk, we mused as we transported them to their new home, what a tale they would tell (Fig. 5.6).

Running a Boat

The process of 'running a boat' (making a collective meal) required as many persons who could contribute something, however small, to donate what they had to the preparation of the meal. One contributor would supply the rice, another the meat ('the salt thing'); a few ackees (a

Jamaican vegetable); an ounce of butter. Somebody would prepare the fire; another would provide the pots. Together we would share in the preparation of the meal. In this way, everybody would be able to have a meal, something to eat in times of scarcity. During the theatre construction process, since many patients were involved in the process of creation of the building, I was able to negotiate with the hospital kitchen to supply the raw materials for their food to the Cultural Therapy Centre and the team members would add these supplies to what was brought by others to the table to 'run the boat.' We cooked food for everybody who was involved in building this theatre. The theatre, a multi-purpose one, was being built from material donated by several firms and individuals and was able to accommodate approximately 1500 persons, when the pageant opened on August 30, 1978.

One of the most remarkable aspects of the creation of *Madnificent Irations* was the productive energy generated during the process of building the theatre. Patients and workers turned up almost magically, on a daily basis, to help to carry out the numerous tasks required for its completion. Deep holes were dug to receive the disused telegraph poles donated by the Jamaica Power Service that served as the foundation pillars of the theatre. Men and women formed a living chain to transport the red bricks dug out of abandoned buildings in the hospital to lay the beautiful floor. I worked with the patient teams in lifting the lighting stanchions constructed from galvanized pipe from the welding shed to the theatre to create the stage lighting rigs. My experience as a stage manager in New York, London and Sydney Opera House certainly came in handy in helping to design and construct the lighting and other technical aspects of the theatre. Finally, the theatre was completed, Pat Staniger's design brought to life. The *Jamaica Daily News* of Monday, August 28, 1978 published a photograph of the Garden Theatre with the following caption: 'Staff and patients at the Bellevue Hospital, putting finishing touches to the open air theatre being constructed for the "Bellevue Week" activities which begin on Wednesday…'.

But perhaps one of the most remarkable discoveries was of a patient who turned out to be a talented wood-carver; he spontaneously started sculpting exquisite carvings out of the trunks of the lignum vitae trees. He seemed to just turn up out of the blue, and without seeking permission identified the dried sections of the trees and began to carve the most beautiful African statues. The uncanny resemblance to Nigerian statues I had seen at the office of the Nigerian Ambassador to Jamaica was remarkable. Our patient was an intuitive who had never left the shores of Jamaica, and who was untrained. The carvings were entirely from his imagination (Figs. 5.7 and 5.8).

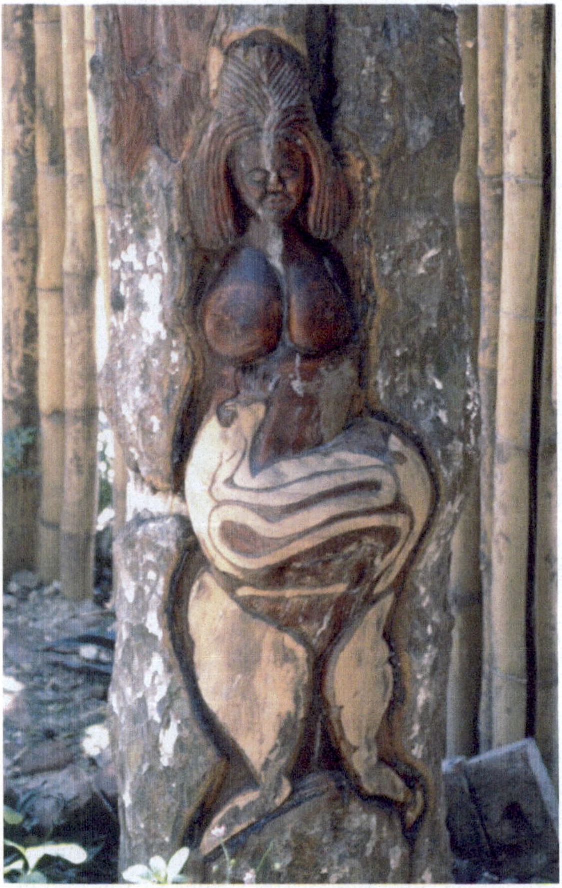

Fig. 5.7 Naturalistic African iconic carving on the trunk of a living lignum vitae tree

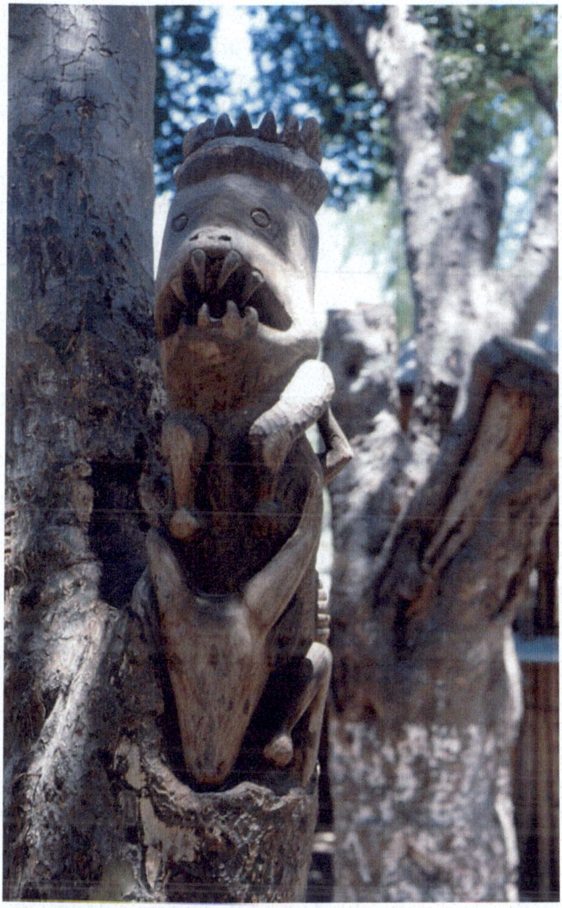

Fig. 5.8 Naturalistic African iconic carving on the truncated branch of a living lignum vitae tree

The Cultural Therapy Program

The initial ethnohistorical Town Hall meetings were held in the established Occupational Therapy Centre of the Bellevue Hospital. However as the script for *Madnificent Irations* emerged, there was a sense of excitement that propelled the workers and patients into building the

Garden Theatre. The 30 psychiatric aides who had been trained at the EMCVPA were drafted by the hospital administration into the Cultural Therapy Team under the leadership of registered nursing sister Neila Johnson. They began developing the cultural therapy program for the hospital. A building in the hospital compound was selected to house this new team, which was structured exactly like a conventional psychiatric ward, with a consultant psychiatrist, medical officer, charge nurse, registered nurses and the assistant nurses and psychiatric aides who were trained in the cultural arts program.

The Morning Session

The team began operating on two shifts, between 7 a.m. and 11 p.m. It was the initial intention to have the Centre operate on a 24-hour basis, as it was recognized that many mentally ill people have difficulty sleeping at night, and that much effective therapy can be accomplished in the early hours of the morning in the appropriate type of facility. In the face of mounting conflicts with senior nursing management over this, the compromise was that the program, divided into morning and afternoon sessions, would end at 11 p.m. This disused building was situated between the site for the Garden Theatre and the established thriving 40-bed Rehabilitation Unit on the north-eastern corner of the hospital compound. The Cultural Therapy Team took charge and refurbished this building as the Cultural Therapy Centre and the three units—the Rehabilitation Unit, the Cultural Therapy Centre, and the Garden Theatre—began to operate as a single functional Service under my leadership and guidance. Patients, nurses, aides, and other medical staff would meet daily to discuss the assignments for the activities of each day.

The psychiatric aides of the Cultural Therapy Team were assigned to the two working shifts, the first between 7 a.m. and 3 p.m. and the second between 3 p.m. and 11 p.m., and these became the operational times of the Cultural Therapy Centre and the Garden Theatre. The two areas became the operational space for the Service. The psychiatric aides on the morning shift would be assigned to visit each of the 25 wards of the hospital and select patients eligible for participating in the cultural therapy program. These selected patients would then be brought by the nurses and aides from their residential wards to assemble in the Garden Theatre area where they would participate in a wide variety of structured dance, drama and creative arts activities led by assigned psychiatric aides.

In this way, the Cultural Therapy Team organized to get hundreds of long-stay patients with severe enduring mental illness and their nurses to leave their residential ward and travel to the other side of the hospital to participate in the cultural therapy activities. The collective process of cultural therapy involved the syncretic blend of large group psychotherapy with the elements and essence of cultural activities such as psychohistoriography, the oral tradition, the use of the circle, folk traditions, storytelling, poetry, arts, crafts, music, dance, and theatre [14]. The process was combined in an eclectic manner with conventional psychopharmacology, and culturally sensitive counseling and psychotherapy.

Centering was a daily warm-up cultural therapy exercise which would be held before each major activity session. Borrowed from the warm-up process utilized by dramatists, dancers, and athletes, the purpose of this process was to provide therapy in itself by stimulating physical exercise, removing inhibitions, facilitating self-confidence, and to encourage collective activity (Fig. 5.9).

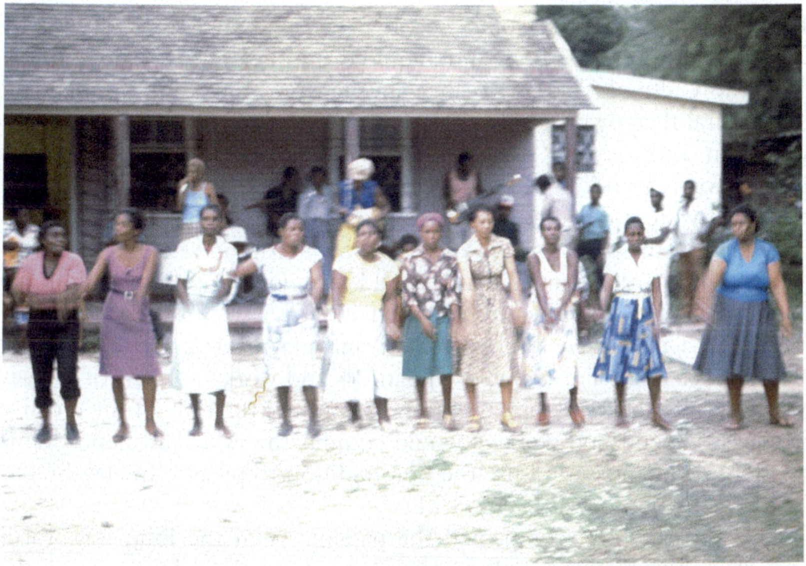

Fig. 5.9 Patients from the long-stay wards and staff, participating in dance therapy centering activities at the morning sessions of the cultural therapy program

The process also sensitized and prepared participants for the rigorous therapeutic activities to follow. Each centering exercise was 5 to 20 minutes long.

Standing in a circle and led by a centering instructor the process would comprise a variety of physical stretching, deep breathing and relaxation exercises, mime, singing, and dance routines. All centering exercises would vary in complexity and would be taken by users and carers. Philosophically, this process draws on the hypnotic mental and physical processes found in other similar cultural processes such as yoga, tai chi, and karate. At lunchtime, these patients would be returned to their respective wards for their mid-day meal. This cultural therapy mobilization program that affected the entire hospital continued in the afternoons, when the major activity would be playmaking and rehearsals, where the patients would participate both as performers in the playmaking and as an audience for the process.

The Afternoon Session

This afternoon sessions would be organized and structured differently from the morning sessions and required another level of functioning from the Cultural Therapy Team. The newly formed Irations Band of the cultural therapy process would play an important central role in these afternoon and evening sessions. There would be rehearsals for plays already written and staged, and collaborative preparation of new pageants that were still being developed (Fig. 5.10).

Not all of the patients who came for the afternoon sessions would be engaged in active playmaking and would form part of the large audience that participated in these afternoon activities they were witnessing. They were placed in graded levels of dance and playmaking activities taking place on the stage. For many, both patients and workers, levels of literacy were low and hence the oral tradition constituted the bulk of the creative activities. Patients and workers would commit the new dance and drama creations to memory, and use the oral tradition to propel the day-by-day creative activities forward (Fig. 5.11).

The nurses who accompanied the patients from the long-stay wards were also obliged to make observations about the clinical progress of the patients under their care, and to record them in the patients' case notes. The cultural therapy mobilization program was thus able to activate patients and workers from the entire hospital and to generate a seminal

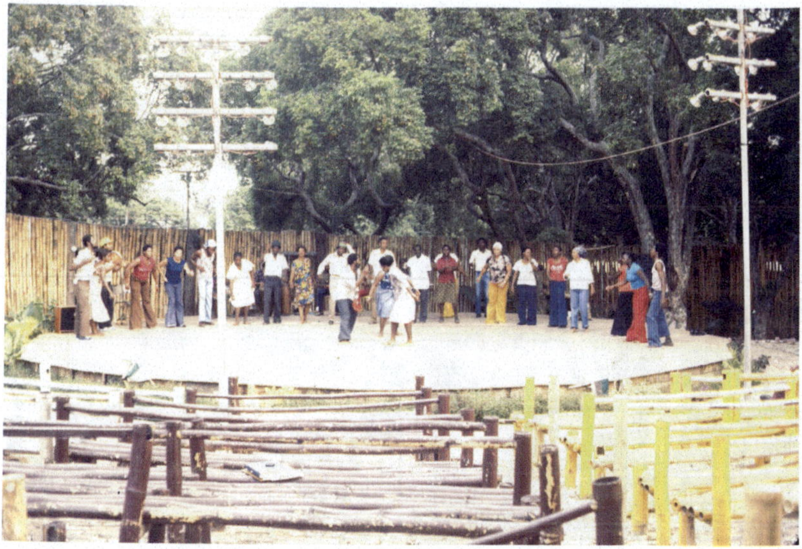

Fig. 5.10 *Madnificent Irations* cast in rehearsal at the Garden Theatre, August 1978

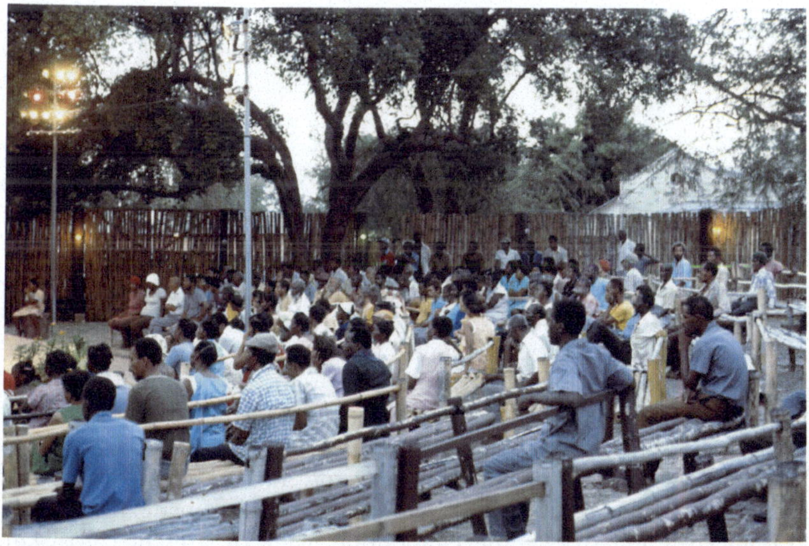

Fig. 5.11 Patients from the long-stay wards attending the afternoon sessions of the cultural therapy program at the Garden Theatre

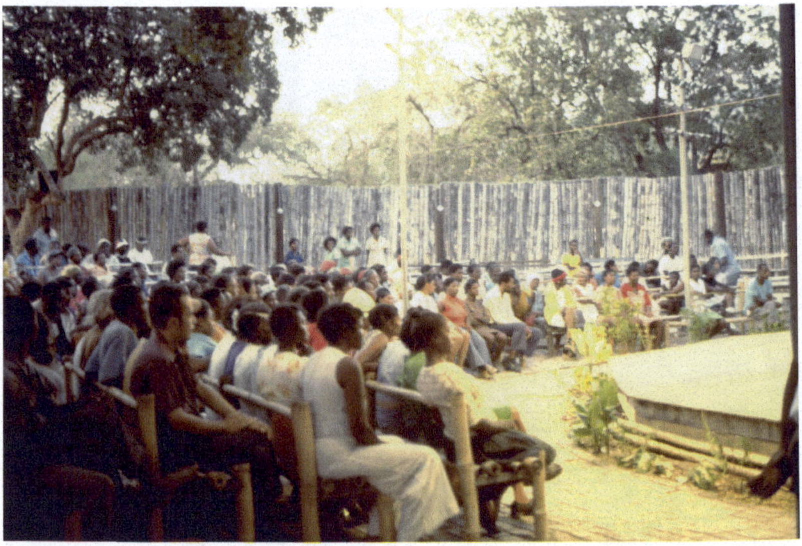

Fig. 5.12 Patients from the long-stay wards attending cultural therapy sessions in the afternoon at the Garden Theatre

new rehabilitative thrust for the institution, converting the passive warehousing hitherto characteristic of the hospital into a dynamic process of rehabilitation (Fig. 5.12).

The Irations Band

The Rastafarian drums (often called harps by the Rastafari) were the central focus of the musical rhythm base of *Madnificent Irations* and featured throughout the pageant. The Rastafari drum trio consisted of a single, central, low-pitched 'thunder' drum, which provided the rhythmic bassline. This was accompanied by the three mid-range 'fundeh' drums, with slack drum heads, and the high-pitched 'repeater' or 'kete' drum, with a tighter drum head, which, under the expert attention of the kete drummer, provided an exquisite syncopated range of melodies. Together, they provided a rich melange of conversational drumming. The congo drum, the 'shaka' or homemade shaker made from a dry coconut shell and stones, the tambourine made of stretched goatskin, and the scraper made from a bamboo joint and a wooden rod provided

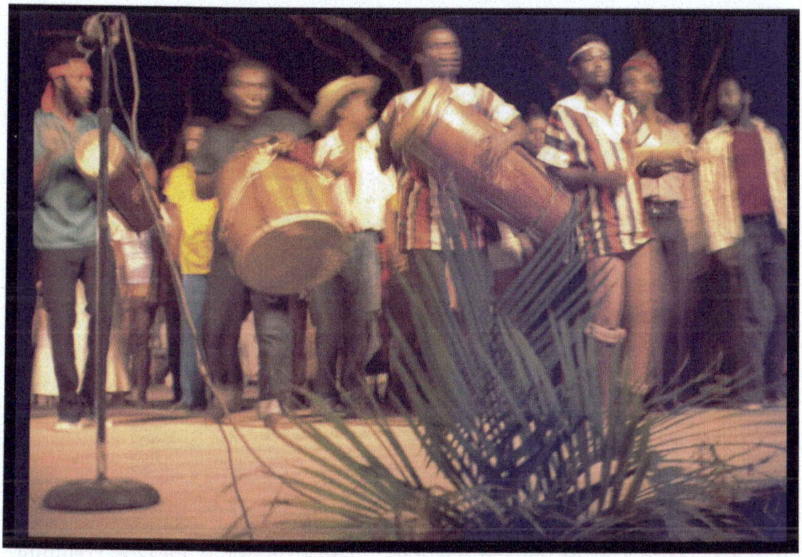

Fig. 5.13 The Rastafari drum ensemble of the Irations Band, comprising the 'fundeh' (front row, left) the 'thunder' (second from left), the African congo (third from left), and the bamboo scraper (extreme right). The kete drum is played while seated and is not shown in this photograph

additional percussive elements. All the drummers were patients and staff of the hospital and the kete drummer was a singularly talented Rastafari patient who entranced listeners with his rhythmic syncopated transitions. The drums were all made locally by a team under the direction of skilled drum maker Phillip Supersad [16], who had interned with the Cultural Therapy Centre while still a student at the EMCVPA (Fig. 5.13).

Some of Jamaica's most talented musicians have been patients of Bellevue throughout its history. When the hospital functioned as a human warehouse, their musical talent was completely buried and abandoned. However, as the theatre emerged these talented musicians also emerged from the woodwork of the hospital, at first timidly, and then more confidently, requesting, demanding musical instruments with which to exercise their talent, and an opportunity to use their skills and to show off their talents. One of the most remarkable talents to emerge was trombonist Eleazor 'Trummie' Beckford, trained at the Alpha

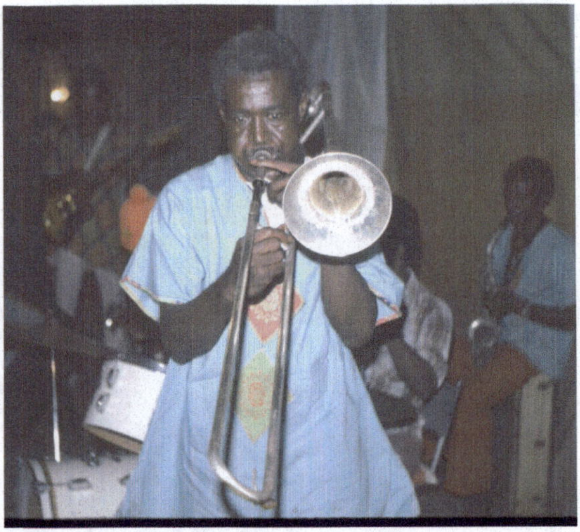

Fig. 5.14 Musicians of the Irations Band, with trombonist Eleazor 'Trummie' Beckford in the foreground

Academy, and incarcerated in Bellevue for almost his entire life. He had no known family, and the hospital became his home and the Irations Band his workplace (Fig. 5.14).

When world-famous trombonist Don Drummond [17] was a patient at Bellevue in the 1960s Beckford and Drummond were cellmates. I secured a trombone for Trummie from Captain Wade of the Jamaica Defence Force band; I then purchased the materials to make the set of Rastafari fundeh, repeater and kete drums which we made, and overnight the Irations Band was formed! One of the sanitation workers employed by the hospital turned up with his saxophone and homemade flute and joined the band.

The Singers and Dancers

It was as if the music was a magnet to the surrounding inner-city Kingston communities as well, and a number of talented young musicians, men and women, all self-trained who lived in nearby communities, started showing up at the Cultural Therapy Centre every day, and soon became part of the Irations Band. Another great find was a patient with

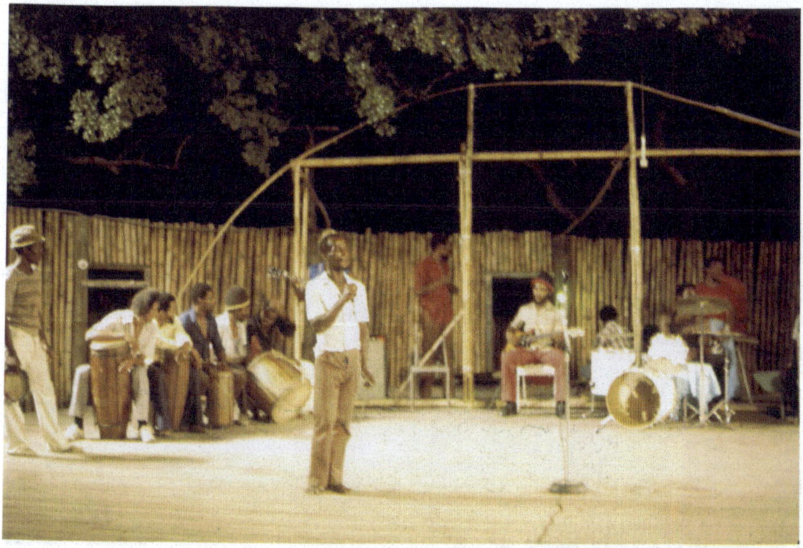

Fig. 5.15 The patient with the beautiful singing voice, dubbed 'song-bird' by the Irations Band; his rendition of Sam Cooke's *Wonderful World* was perfection

a 'song-bird' singing voice who could imitate the songs of the famous African American singer of the 1960s to perfection. 'Sam Cook', as this patient became known, was attracted to the Irations Band like a moth to a light, and became an inseparable and valuable member of the band (Fig. 5.15).

The singers and dancers who made up the largest numbers of performers consisted of male and female patients from the long-stay wards of the hospital, along with a few of the nursing aides. The stirring performances that these so-called chronic mad people put on consistently, day after day, night after night, soon challenged the perception of 'madness' on the part of the hospital staff, other patients and the wider community [18] (Fig. 5.16).

Evening Entertainment at the Garden Theatre

Perhaps the most remarkable aspect of the daily life of the Cultural Therapy Centre was the period after five o'clock in the afternoon, as day became night. Most people in the surrounding communities were just

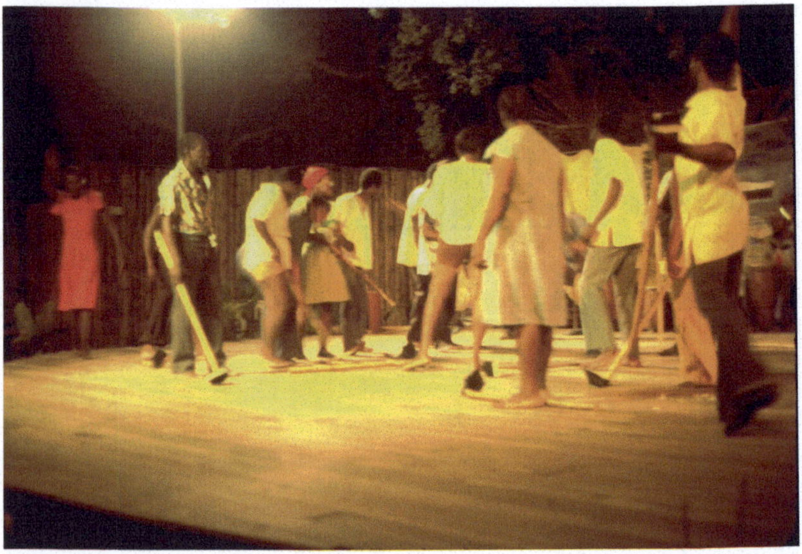

Fig. 5.16 Patient singers and dancers: The conventional conception of 'chronic' madness was hopelessness, helplessness, and characterological deterioration that beggared the imagination. *Madnificent Irations* put paid to those notions once and for all and was the turning point in the decolonization of madness in Jamaica and the dawn of a new direction for psychiatry in the region

coming home from work and were looking for some form of cultural activity and entertainment. Many of the hospital workers were just completing their shift or had finished work for the day and were looking to play a game of dominos, to hold a beer or just to 'cool off' before going home. And what became evident to the administration of the hospital was that many of their patients were night people and were all looking for activity at this time of day. It was during the evening that the Garden Theatre became a cultural engagement center that forged a link between the surrounding community, the hospital workers, and the patients, many of whom found solace in the night.

All parts of the equation worked syncretically for peace, stability, and cultural engagement. This part of Kingston city in the late 1970s was like a war zone, as the political gangs squared off against each other with high caliber weaponry. But the Bellevue Garden Theatre became a remarkable center of tranquility and peace. The evolution took place naturally. By mutual agreement of the community, no guns were allowed in the Garden Theatre. The JLP constituents from Paradise Street and adjoining areas in the West sat peacefully with their PNP neighbors from Brown's Town in the North and Dunkirk and Rockfort in the East. The Cultural Therapy Team would provide food and drink for a small charge from their entrepreneurial tuck shop, and the cultural therapy workers on duty would keep a watchful clinical eye over the patients who came and participated in all the activities of the evening. The filling or meat of the evening sandwich came from the community cultural therapy program that went on through the evening until after 11 p.m. The Irations Band would provide the musical backing and anybody from the audience could come up on the stage to exercise their talent and perform for the people who were assembled. Thus, many talented singers, musicians, poets, and dramatists were allowed a time on the stage to 'bus', as it was called colloquially. To 'bus' (burst) meant to make a debut in live performance on stage or on a microphone and that one had an opportunity to expose one's talent; to perform to a live audience; to be in charge of the microphone for a period of time. Depending on how the eager new performer aiming to 'bus' was received by the audience would dictate how much time they would have on the stage with the microphone in hand. The opportunity gave one an opportunity to impress a music producer who might be quietly present in the audience, and who might invite you to his recording studio to 'cut a tune.'

The evenings were successful, enjoyable, and productive for all concerned; they very quickly began to exercise a powerful 'political' effect on the entire community. This was positive and rewarding for some, and extremely threatening for others. The Garden Theatre became a 'safe place' for community residents from all neighboring districts, without fear of conflict generated by political party labels.

The community visitors were of all ages: children, adolescents, young, and old adults. All were welcome, and all felt comfortable to participate within the space of the mental hospital. Occasionally, the Garden Theatre was rented out by a performing group for their own private production and performance. The Sistren Theatre Collective was a popular theatre organization of women who would sometimes perform one of their productions at the theatre. On other occasions, well-known internationally famous Jamaican entertainers and artistes such as Mutabaruka and Jean

'Binta' Breeze would stop by in the evening and perform for the assembled audience. *Madnificent Irations* had 'flipped' madness in the social psyche of the Jamaican people, making the Bellevue Garden Theatre the revolutionary 'safe place' for Jamaican cultural and political reasonings.

Bibliography

1. Hickling FW (1985) Poem "Westminster System" (Unpublished).
2. Hickling FW (1975) *The Establishment of Rehabilitation Service at Bellevue Mental Hospital, Jamaica and an Analysis of the First Six Months of that Service*, Doctoral Thesis, Psychiatry Department, University of the West Indies.
3. Hickling FW and Gibson R (2005) The History of Caribbean Psychiatry. In F Hickling, E Sorel (Eds.), *Images of Psychiatry*. Kingston: Stephenson's Litho Press Ltd.
4. Hickling-Hudson A (2011) Postcolonialism, Hybridity and Transferability: The Contribution of Pamela O'Gorman to Music Education in the Caribbean. *Caribbean Journal of Education, 1 & 2*, 36–55.
5. *The Star*, June 30 1977.
6. Hamilton B (1977) New Get-Well Techniques at Bellevue—Using Culture to Help the Mentally Ill. *Jamaica Daily News*, July 5.
7. Jones M (1968) *Social Psychiatry in Practice: The Idea of a Therapeutic Community*. Harmondsworth, Middlesex: Penguin.
8. Brodber E (1983) Oral Sources and the Creation of Social History in the Caribbean. *Jamaica Journal, 16*(4), 2–8.
9. Miller P (1992) The Tavistock Mission: A Review Essay. *Human Relations, 45*(4), 411–426.
10. Nettleford R, Stone C (1977) *Worker Participation*. Kingston: Government of Jamaica Printer.
11. Manley M (1974) *The Politics of Change: A Jamaican Testament*. London: Andre Deutsch.
12. Barnett L (1975) Report of a Commission of Enquiry into the Attempted Outbreak from the St. Catherine District Prison, Jamaica, on December 20, 1974. Jamaica Government Report.
13. Gleaner Online (2015) Revisiting Green Bay. The Killings of 1978. A Gleaner Online Special. http://digjamaica.com/m/blog/a-moment-in-history-the-green-bay-massacre/.
14. Levy H (1978) What Goes on at Bellevue? *Jamaica Daily News*, Wednesday, August 2.
15. Bennett W, Bennett H (2011) *The Jamaican Theatre: Highlights of the Performing Arts in the Twentieth Century*. Kingston: University of the West Indies Press.

16. Cooke M (2009) Drumming Stays with Supersad. *The Jamaica Gleaner*, Sunday, July 20.
17. Augustyn H (2013) *Don Drummond: The Genius and Tragedy of the World's Greatest Trombonist*. Jefferson, NC: McFarland.
18. Hickling FW (1989) Sociodrama in the Rehabilitation of Chronic Mental Illness. *Hospital and Community Psychiatry*, *40*, 402–406.

CHAPTER 6

Psychohistoriographic Cultural Therapy: The Technique

Him throw de crumbs gi we again
'Come on Blackie, take the reins'
while him still own all de factory
An de lan an sugar canes. [1]

The use of culture as an instrument for education, consciousness-raising, and demystification, as well as using entertainment as a tool through which the peoples of the world have mounted the struggle for freedom, land, and better working conditions, has existed for centuries. This has been rediscovered and titled people's or popular theatre [2] in recent years and combines the use of dialect, folk poetry, drama, dance, music, and song to mobilize people to utilize their creative cultural energy in the struggle against racism and oppression, and in the fight for rights, justice, and better conditions. Ross Kidd [3] described the process as 'the people's medium, drawing on their skills and creativity, expressing their concerns and analysis, [and] reinforc[ing] the growth of identity and self-confidence'. Iconic Brazilian educator and philosopher Paulo Freire [4, 5] emphasized the idea of education as cultural action, and that the liberation from oppression requires collective struggle. The transformation of any society requires the development of revolutionary consciousness and the mobilization of a culture of creativity. The process, as Kidd describes, must 'mirror reality,' must lend itself to a dialectical world view, demystifying the notion of social change as a 'neutral

F. W. Hickling, *Decolonization of Psychiatry in Jamaica*,
https://doi.org/10.1007/978-3-030-48489-7_6

technical process' and must challenge insightful understanding of social oppression and enslavement, demanding change by active participation.

The development of an active popular theatre movement in Jamaica intensified in the decade of the 1970s, building on the blueprint of Marcus Garvey and Edelweiss Park in Kingston in the early 1910s. Garvey insisted that Black Jamaicans must provide an arena for their creative expression in drama, music, and poetry. Edelweiss Park [6] provided that opportunity, where Jamaican artists and performers were allowed to express their creativity on a regular basis and at the same time provide the basis for regular paid employment in the performing arts. In the context of colonial Jamaica at the turn of the century, this was revolutionary activity and laid the basis for the development of contemporary theatre. Popular performers such as Louise Bennett, Ranny Williams, Bim and Bam, laid the early foundation. By the early 1970s, the Jamaican cultural scene was exploding [7] with the reggae music of Bob Marley, Peter Tosh, and countless others, and in the theatrical world, Trevor Rhone, Lloyd Reckord, and Rex Nettleford were beginning to leave their mark. The 1970s saw a plethora of new talent arising, and the popular theatre trend produced a wave of performing groups which were based in socio-political organizations of the time, always reflecting a class position. The Sistren Theatre Collective emerged from a political collective of Jamaican working women. The Bellevue Cultural Team and the Gun Court Theatre Movement emerged from the island's custodial institutions, and from the newly formed Edna Manley Cultural Training Centre emerged the Graduate Theatre Company, later to become known as the Groundwork Theatre Company. This arm of the popular theatre movement had the essential characteristic of being supported financially by governmental and non-governmental organizations. Simultaneously, self-sustaining theatre for profit began to emerge with producers such as Ralph Holness, Ed Wallace, and Hugh King leading the way, giving birth to popular playwriting and performing talents such as Balfour Anderson, Patrick Brown, and Oliver Samuels. This challenged the traditional performance giants such as the Little Theatre Movement, the National Dance Theatre Company (NDTC), and the government-sponsored Jamaica Festival.

The idea of creating pageants to depict the historical origin of groups and organizations came early in my life. I was a youthful schoolboy when my mother, who was a gifted classical pianist and music teacher, wrote a historical pageant—*Life More Abundant*—to commemorate the history of the St. Andrew High School for Girls in the mid-1950s. Kathleen Bond-Hickling trained in classical piano at the Royal Academy of Music in London in the early 1930s and returned to Jamaica to set up the Kathleen Bond School for classical piano in Kingston in 1935. Nearly fifty years later she received the Silver Musgrave Medal from the Institute of Jamaica for her contribution to the development of music in Jamaica. As the son of this well-known and established Jamaican music teacher, I grew up in a musical family and was, from an early age, exposed to all types of music and the theatre. I have been involved in theatre productions since leaving Wolmer's High School for Boys in 1961, having been active in the school's drama club. I started working with performers with the Jamaica Festival Movement in the early 1960s, such as Tommy McCook and the Skatalites Band, Hortense Ellis, Toots and the Maytals, and many other well-known popular Jamaican artistes. I became the stage manager for the NDTC in 1962 and remained in that capacity until 1977 when I launched out into poetry and playwriting, entertainment production, and performance direction. In my formative years in the theatre in Jamaica, I gained expertise at home and abroad in the production and management of stage performances. This experience also provided me with first-hand knowledge of the architecture of theatres and performing centers, all of which provided the foundations for the creation of *Madnificent Irations* and building the Bellevue Hospital Garden Theatre.

While the theatre was being constructed, the first Bellevue pageant, *Madnificent Irations*, was taking shape. The script reflected the many themes and trends that emerged from the ethnohistorical meetings. The script was written in the Jamaican free-verse style called dub poetry, similar to the style of *Explanitations*, which I had written some months before for the Third World Band. I have described in the chapter titled 'Catalyzing Creativity', in my book jointly edited with Eliot Sorel, Professor of Psychiatry and Public Health at George Washington University, how the rudimentary elements of the cultural therapy process originated in a workshop that I held with the young and extremely talented reggae band Third World, in 1977 [8]. The collaboration of a psychiatrist with the band served to challenge the stigma that surrounded psychiatry and mental health, and to identify clearly my dual role and status as psychiatrist and artistic director in the workshop process. In that article, I described the development program for the band, which incorporated a daily didactic one-hour group session with the band members, conducted on conventional psychotherapeutic principles, using free association techniques, personal and historical self-disclosure, and the management of group transference relationships. The meetings focused on power relationships and dynamics within the group, including the musicians and the management and technical team. Emerging from these group meetings, I completed an artistic and creative analysis and outlined the development of a new type of show, based on the syncretic concept of the band itself, the Third World cultural and historical dynamic, and the examination of the very idea of the Third World Man. This work was the first of its kind in Jamaica and the world that incorporated dub poetry, Rastafari culture, and reggae music into a coherent script, with active characters and a story line. *Explanitations*, as the show was called, was a smash hit, broke every box-office record in Jamaica, and soon Third World was to achieve international stardom.

Jamaican psychiatrists of the 1970s were having to deal increasingly with young Jamaicans, particularly males, brought in for evaluation after they started to smoke ganja (cannabis), grow their hair in 'dreadlocks,' adopt a vegetarian lifestyle, and follow the Rastafarian movement. Many of these young people who were undergoing conversion to Rastafari were often regarded by their parents and communities as exhibiting insanity brought on by the ritual smoking of ganja, and many had been diagnosed by psychiatrists as having a cannabis psychosis. A young adult struggling to separate from a family by joining a new religion is not a new clinical situation. In the Jamaican context, clinicians often refer to the transforming process as the 'Rastoid' phenomenon, which must be distinguished from the process of transformation that is catalyzed by significant psychopathology [9].

'Catalyzing Creativity' also described the birth of psychohistoriographic cultural therapy at the Bellevue Hospital in 1978. The process was also described in greater detail in my book *Psychohistoriography*, published in 2007 [10]. The collective process of cultural therapy involved the syncretic blend of large group psychotherapy with the elements and essence of cultural activities of psychohistoriography: the oral tradition, the use of the circle, folk traditions, storytelling, poetry, arts, crafts, music, dance, and theatre. The sociodrama process emerged with the creation of *Madnificent Irations* as progressing through five distinct stages, with stages 1–3 described in this chapter and stages 4 and 5 in Chapter 7. Stage 1 is the *phase of the ethnohistorical meetings and the psychohistoriographic analysis*. Stage 2 is the *phase of creation of the script*.

Stage 3 is the *phase of staging and production*. Stage 4 is the *phase of performance*, while Stage 5 is the *phase of evaluation*.

Stage 1: The Ethnohistorical Meetings and the Psychohistoriographic Analysis

As part of the rehabilitation transformation process that I was introducing at the mental hospital, I started a series of monthly Town Hall meetings with the staff and patients of the hospital. This was an adaptation of the *therapeutic community process* that had been established by Maxwell Jones in the UK. This period witnessed the creation of the bulwark of my knowledge and experience that catapulted me into the rehabilitation and deinstitutionalization process at Bellevue Hospital later in that decade. The ethnohistorical meetings consisted of groups of staff and patients up to three hundred in number. Prior to this, patients only came in contact with staff in the very restricted environments of the custodial wards and rarely had an opportunity to discuss their ideas and concerns with the staff or indeed, themselves. The therapeutic group meetings that were introduced as a daily activity in the 24 hospital wards began to facilitate open therapeutic discussions between staff and patients, as part of an attempt to flatten the severe hierarchical operational power structure of the functional units. A nominated chairperson would lead each group and would incorporate cultural activities such as ring games, storytelling, and improvisation. These groups were held on a daily basis and became part of the psychotherapeutic functions of this psychiatric hospital.

The Town Hall or ethnohistorical meetings were intended to provide a forum to facilitate mutual understanding of the 'madness' that had led the patients to be admitted and which the staff was attempting to treat. They also included discussions and activities that were audio- and/or videotaped at specific times to record the folk and historical material generated by the process. The meetings were held monthly in the Occupational Therapy Centre, which was the only physical location in the hospital at the time that could accommodate this large a number of people. Each meeting was attended by patients and staff, including senior administrators, doctors and nurses, psychiatric aides, and domestic and ancillary workers. Each meeting was tape-recorded and the discussions analyzed to determine the major themes that emerged, and to note the changing attitudes and perceptions of the staff. One patient, known as 'Mackie,' described with chilling detail how the nurses used to subdue patients with sheets and towels, often choking them almost to the point of asphyxiation. Mackie's openly verbalized recollections triggered a howl of protest from the nursing staff who were present. The protest was not concerned with the accuracy of his tales. The nurses were more concerned that the ethnohistorical meetings were allowing the patients an opportunity to verbalize their anger toward the all-powerful nursing staff, in an environment when the patients could not be forcibly silenced, and were thereby eroding what the nurses perceived as the authority base of the nursing staff for immediate and future control of the patients in the hospital. The moderator had the difficult task of facilitating the cathartic discussion of the dialectics of custodialization versus freedom and coercion versus voluntary acceptance of treatment.

Out of the ethnohistorical meetings grew the process of psychohistoriography, which, since transforming the process of insight at Bellevue Hospital, has become a fundamental analytic methodology of cultural therapy, and has been applied to widely differing areas in psychiatry and psychology especially in the psychotherapeutic treatment of diverse racial groups [10–12]. The technique of psychohistoriography was adapted from the process of historiography, the latter being a methodology that had been used by historians to analyze historical documents to determine a society's outlook, ideology, and benefits, and to identify the dynamics and social forces that drive change. I had come across the concept while I was a physician-intern at the University Hospital of the West Indies, caring for famous Caribbean historian Elsa Goveia in the period prior to her death. Our discussions while she was a patient led me to read her seminal work *A Study on the Historiography of the British West Indies* (1956) [13], which had become a central work in the shaping of historical analysis at the University of the West Indies. In her introduction, she quoted Carl Becker's 1938 definition of historiography as 'a phase of intellectual history...which records what men have at different times known and believed about the past, the use they have made in the service of their interests and aspirations, of their knowledge and beliefs, and the underlying presuppositions which made their knowledge seem to them relevant and their beliefs seem to them true' [14].

Historians have used historiography to analyze the writings of historians in terms of their outlook, ideology, and beliefs in order to identify the changes in a given society. Often, there have existed conflicting views between historians and psychiatrists as the latter have tended to make causal (biological) explorations, whereas historians have tended to address themselves to the understanding of actual experiences in all their detail. Karl Jaspers suggested that sciences that include both fields of enquiry, such as psychopathology and history, work together for their mutual advancement [15]. He described the investigation of psychopathological phenomena in society and in history as being of importance for attaining a realistic perspective on our total human reality. He proposed that the psychiatrist must always prepare a thorough social anamnesis, establishing where patients have come from and what life experiences and influences they have been subject to. For therapy to progress and change to take place, patients too must internalize these insights in order to facilitate transformation, problem-solving and reality testing and overcome the forces that inhibit action. In the process they will learn to master the anxieties that attend the pursuit of normal life goals, come to terms with personal limitations and handicaps, while fulfilling themselves to the highest degree of their creative potential.

Psychohistoriography is a postcolonial model of psychoanalysis, developed at Bellevue in the 1970s as a technique for catalyzing insight [16]. I created the neologism *psychohistoriography* as a combined derivation from the word *psyche*, capturing the oral process of the mind as described by Brodber [17], and *historiography*, from the orthodox historical word as defined by Becker and Goveia. Using the *oral tradition* and *historiography*, I created the technique that I called psychohistoriography, which emerged out of the ethnohistorical large group meetings at Bellevue as I struggled to make coherent sense of the stormy, often conflictual discussions of oral history that emerged from the discourse between patients and staff. The psychohistoriographic process that emerged was designed to produce insight into a group situation by analyzing the historical material in a graphic form within a dialectical perspective to identify reality-based themes and trends, to facilitate productivity and change for the individuals and the group, to help underdeveloped and colonized people to debunk myth, and to establish reality as a framework for future action. Following each ethnohistorical meeting, I replayed the audio tapes of the meetings, and on a large sheet of cartridge paper I started to create the first psychohistoriogram that became the foundation for the script of *Madnificent Irations*.

Creating the Psychohistoriogram

The psychohistoriogram was a large chart on which historical, cultural, and behavioral analyses were documented, using material culled from the ethnohistorical meetings; its thematic constructs were based on insights extrapolated by visual inspection and intuitive analysis. The initial psychohistoriogram was developed over a period of weeks, as the verbal historical material was charted as the dialectical discussions emerged. In 1979, when I was writing up the process of the creation of the pageant and the method of creating the psychohistoriogram, a graphic designer—Howard Salmon—using my original diagram, created four separate charts, to illustrate how the psychohistoriogram was created and how it facilitated the psychohistoriographic analysis that subsequently generated the script [10]. Those four charts were reconstructed facsimiles that were designed to clarify and simplify the overall chart that is presented here (Fig. 6.1).

The graphic matrices provided the template on which the historical anecdotes from the ethnohistorical discussions were recorded. This was followed by the historical analysis that produced the thematic constructs of the script, which in turn catalyzed the creation of the scripted lines of the drama, and the poems and songs that buttressed the emerging pageant. The process is described below. The four charts [10] represented a breakdown of the process for simplification, which in reality was a breakdown of one composite overall master psychohistoriogram. The process of creating the psychohistoriogram was as follows.

Establishing the Graphic Matrices

(a) The Timeline

Using a large chart, the two-dimensional representation and analysis began by creating a horizontal line across the center of the chart (Fig. 6.1) constituting the timeline or time continuum. In the creation of the *Madnificent Irations* psychohistoriogram, the worker ethnohistorical meetings established the period of history that best represented the historical antecedents of madness in Jamaica. The meeting participants decided that the historical period before the arrival of Christopher Columbus would be the starting point of the analysis and the initial year starting the millennium—year 1000—would be charted at the extreme

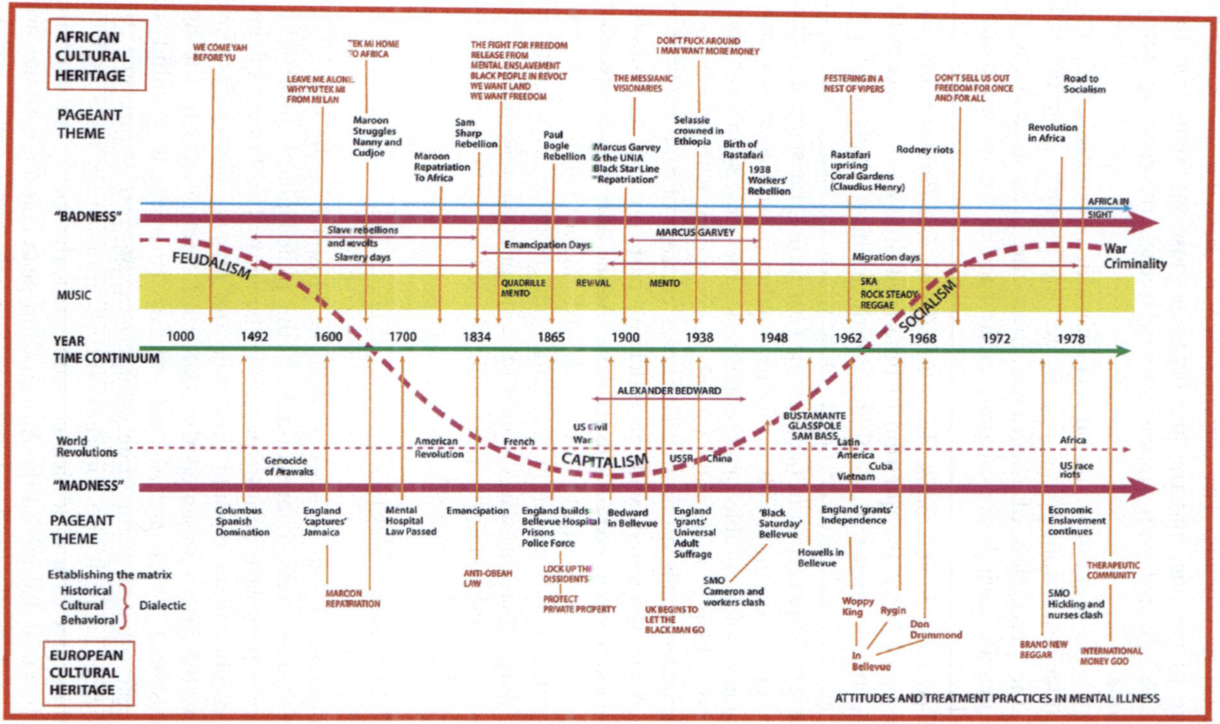

Fig. 6.1 Psychohistoriogram for the *Madnificent Irations* sociopoem showing timeline, dialectical antipodes, and vertical theme lines with analytic insights at either end

left edge of the timeline. The current year was charted at the extreme right edge of the line, and the line between those two points on the chart was subdivided with equidistant points each representing equal time periods.

By drawing a horizontal line on a chalkboard, to represent the time period under discussion, I was able to get the group's attention and broaden the perception of themselves from the present moment in time, to include their historical past, as far back as we wished to go, collectively.

I recalled John Mbiti's book *African Religions and Philosophy* [18] in which he opined that the question of time is of little or no concern to African peoples in their traditional life. For them, life is simply a composition of events which have occurred, those which are taking place now, and those which are certain to occur in the near future. He suggested that what is certain to occur, or falls within the rhythm of natural phenomena, is the category of inevitable or potential time, the most significant consequence of which is a two-dimensional phenomenon, with a long past, a present, and virtually no future. The linear concept of time in Western thought, Mbiti suggested, with an indefinite past, present, and infinite future, is largely foreign to African thinking. Actual time is therefore what is present and what is past. It moves 'backward' rather than 'forward,' and people set their minds not on future things, but chiefly on what has taken place. I thought that this was a wonderful concept applicable to descendants of Africans enslaved in the West, which I tried to incorporate into the concept of the psychohistoriogram.

(b) The Dialectical Matrix

The psychohistoriographic work at Bellevue Hospital in the late 1970s represented a syncretic connection with the philosophical understanding of these post-slave African people in Jamaica. The horizontal line on the chalkboard represented time *past and present*. The space above and below the line represented the *dialectical* determinants of the history represented by the *psychological anecdotes* emerging from minds of these people situated in the large group *ethnohistorical* discussion [10]. All the themes brought into conscious verbalizations at the meeting were expressed in three clear dialectical continua: first, the social class dialectic; second, the racial dialectic of the African/European cultural heritage; and third, the madness/badness dialectic of violent behavior in which violence associated with social dissent and penalized by referral to the prison system was contrasted with abnormal ideas and behavior (see previous chapter). These three dialectical antipodes became the basis of a diagrammatic psychohistoriographic analytic scheme. By representing these dialectical antipodes as continuous lines of force which exist in time, the psychohistoriogram set up a two-dimensional spatial matrix on which to fit all the historical perceptions and anecdotes made at the ethnohistorical meeting which could then be analyzed for form and content.

The conventional continuum often used in dialectical analysis concerns social class. The racial/class dialectical matrices were merged with the madness/badness matrix used to develop *Madnificent Irations*. These cross the timeline at right angles and are positioned at the left-hand side of the chart. The African cultural heritage/lower social class antipode was represented in the upper left-hand corner of the chart, and the designated European cultural heritage/upper social class antipode in the lower left-hand corner. For the purposes of the *Madnificent Irations* psychohistoriogram, the African cultural heritage antipode was coterminous with the lower social class antipode as slavery *ipso facto* positioned all Africans relocated to Jamaica in the lowest social class rankings [19]. The legacy of slavery was a social structure where race and class were coterminous [20]. Similarly, by definition in the period of slavery, European cultural heritage was *ipso facto* coterminous with upper social class. The blank psychohistoriogram matrix was then complete and was ready to receive historical data [10].

Establishing Historical Material

As Senior Medical Officer (SMO) and moderator/analyst of these meetings, I ensured that the discussion also took into consideration the 'politics of decolonization' in relation to the history of madness in Jamaica. It involved a dialectical interpretation of the worker participation process (see previous chapter), which was a feature of trade union discussions in Jamaica in the mid-1970s. At the first ethnohistorical meeting held at Bellevue Hospital, I invited fifteen of the oldest workers and patients of the hospital to sit in a circle in the middle of the meeting, and to recollect their memories of the hospital as it existed two, three, and four decades before, when it was named the Jamaica Lunatic Asylum. The meetings triggered profound historical insights and challenging conflicts, catalyzed by the face-to-face exchanges between the older nurses, with their more benevolent anecdotal memories, and by the more bellicose and tempestuous patients who were now part of the group discussion. At the ethnohistorical meetings, the group discussed the history of Jamaica, the history of madness in Jamaica, and the history of Bellevue Hospital using the process of free association. Each historical fact was verified by persons within the group and was referenced wherever possible. Once consensus was achieved regarding each historical datum, it was entered on the chart at the point corresponding to the time it occurred and the collectively agreed upon cultural heritage/class position [10]. As many historical facts as possible were discussed by the group and recorded and very soon the chart became filled with consensual historical material. Fitting the stated perceptions into the psychohistoriographic matrix was an exciting and revealing exercise that exposed historical juxtapositions which, by their very existence, questioned erroneously held concepts of causality.

The psychohistoriogram counterposes events of local significance in Jamaica and the hospital with major global political events occurring at that time. Historical events charted below the timeline reflect the European cultural heritage. It also represents a line of force connecting the American, French, Russian, Cuban, Asian, and African-Caribbean revolutions, a period spanning over 200 years. Facts charted above the timeline represent known facts of African resistance to slavery and colonialism, and continue that analysis to the present. These historical events are then represented as lines of force acting at right angles to the time continuum, producing from their synthesis a three-dimensional political/social life force which is depicted by a hatched line across the body of the matrix. The insight gleaned by psychohistoriographic analysis with various groups around the globe over the past thirty years suggests that the European invasion of the Caribbean and the New World in the fifteenth and sixteenth centuries was based on a 'delusion of discovery,' which in turn was based on a 'delusion of white supremacy.' This has been called the 'European delusion' or the 'European psychosis', as discussed in Chapter 1.

The literature of the epidemiology and treatment of mental illness in the indigenous populations of the Caribbean is described in Chapter 2. The pre-colonial paradigm for mental health in this region was *communalism*, which is an indigenous system of government in which independent communes or communities participate in loose federations. This was followed by a period of *extermination and genocide* of the indigenous population by the European colonizers. European powers have been fighting over ownership of the Caribbean for the past five hundred years. Genocide of the indigenous populations of the Americas and the Caribbean, and the establishment of African slavery in the New World were products of the European delusional invasion and colonization. The delusion of capitalism emerged from the plantation economies and industrialization spawned by the European-American psychosis. This hegemonic conflict over control of the New World and the Caribbean has continued until today.

Historical Anecdotes About the Asylum

During the period of slavery in the Caribbean, which extended from the early sixteenth to the mid-nineteenth century, the health of slaves was the responsibility of the slave owners. Between the late seventeenth century and emancipation, a violently mentally ill slave would invariably be executed rather than rehabilitated. Torture of slaves in the West Indies may have surpassed the draconian treatment of the mentally ill in European asylums. It is clear that from the inception of slavery in the Caribbean, the Black slaves could not rely on the efficacy of the facilities provided by the slave master or the colonial government for their health treatment and care. Traditional healing practices became the norm for the slave population of the Caribbean, who also had to rely on their traditional healers for the care of their mental illnesses. Traditional medicine in the Caribbean history of slavery and the practice of Obeah, which was made illegal in Jamaica in 1760 and which is still illegal today, was of paramount importance for African slave mental health. This historical period saw the establishment of the first lunatic asylum in the Anglophone Caribbean, which was part of the Kingston Public Hospital in Jamaica, established in 1776. This asylum was described by Richard Rouse, its warden, as being a 'chamber of horrors' [21] as he reported the appalling conditions of overcrowding, poor sanitation, and torture. His book, *New Light on Dark Deeds* (1860), contained damning evidence of the then physician superintendent's insensitivity to the plight of the patients, and established that the use of forced labor and flogging was condoned at that time. His book related the description of a former inmate, Rosa Henry, that there were many people in the madhouse who died from ill treatment, and her experience of Warder Steele as being very cruel.

She described a blow he gave her with a stick which broke her forehead and reported that the physician superintendent, Dr. Scott, would see the warders beating the patients with sticks but would not interfere.

These historical anecdotes of the asylum and how madness was dealt with were entered on the psychohistoriogram, which focuses on the characters of Jamaican history who were involved in the asylum's history. The space below the timeline reflects the creation of the asylum/mental hospital and the important figures who were recalled in the collective consciousness of the ethnohistorical meeting. Patients such as Alexander Bedward, the religious leader of 1895 and Don Drummond, Jamaica's most celebrated trombonist, who died in the hospital in 1969. The space also includes politicians like Alexander Bustamante and Florizel Glasspole, both involved in the first major trade union conflict at Bellevue in 1946, during which the first politically motivated murder attributable to Jamaica's postcolonial two-party system took place. Coincidentally, Glasspole was present as Jamaica's third Governor-General at the opening night of *Madnificent Irations* and can be seen in the photograph depicted in Fig. 4.1. Also featured in the matrix is the English SMO of the 1940s, regarded as one of the most draconian in living memory; as some of the older staff and patients recalled, he used to patrol the grounds of the asylum at night with his gun [10]. Conversely, the space above the timeline reflects persons and events in Jamaican history who are regarded as villains by the colonial government, but as heroes by the people. By the process of visual inspection, the analyst and the group identify specific clusters of charted historical data, and vertical theme lines and horizontal trend lines are established by group consensus.

The Musical Cultural Timeline

Traditional Jamaican drum types have predominantly African origins. During slavery, drumming was often banned because the Whites were irked by the 'heathen' sound of the drum and feared its power. There are a few basic rhythmic methods used in drumming for both communication (as a speech surrogate or 'talking drum') and entertainment. These methods often included rhythmic codes for the sending and receiving of messages over long distances. There are both iconic and symbolic dimensions to communication within music and dance. Throughout many festivals in Africa, depending on the event being celebrated, drumbeats are used to dictate the type of dance performed by participants.

Drumming played a vital part in the slaves' recreation, in their worship, and in their celebrations; as a result, the drum continues to be important and is at the center of our folk culture. It is in the area of folk music and our traditional folk forms that African derived drums and drumming have retained their supremacy. The drum became the centerpiece of the cultural therapy process at Bellevue Hospital. During the creation of the psychohistoriogram, there was a lively discussion about the development of music and drama in Jamaica. And a signal attempt was made to trace the development of musical genres in Jamaica and their competitive/syncretic relationship with European classical music. This was represented on the psychohistoriogram and played an important role in the selection of folk songs and traditional genres represented in the songs and musical representation in *Madnificent Irations* (Fig. 6.2).

In the Jamaican and Caribbean slave culture, the drum has had multiple purposes, ranging from communication, celebration, war calls, and religion. In entertainment, drums collectively are seen as the foundation of a performance. The rhythmic patterns drive the music, giving it a pulse, providing an undeniable urge to the listener to participate. Religious practices like Revival, Kumina, and Rastafari see drumming

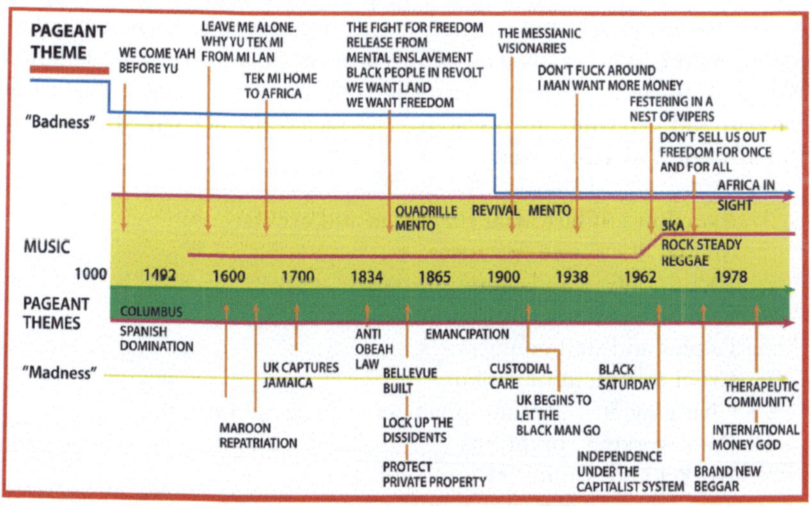

Fig. 6.2 Charting Jamaican musical history on the psychohistoriographic chart in preparation for scripting the *Madnificent Irations* sociopoem

as often establishing a deep connection between man and the spiritual, occasionally placing people in a trance or state of mild hypnosis. Once this happens, the individual, through their mannerism and movements, noticeably mimics the playing of the drums until it stops. Drums were used in *Madnificent Irations* to enhance the learning experience, through combining words with music.

Stage 2: The Creation of the Script

The theme and trend lines are labeled by the group using single words or single phrases which express the participants' perceptions of the theme or the trend. Trend lines can only have one label (on the right-hand side of the chart, but the themes can have labels either at the top or at the bottom of the chart representing the class perceptions of the historical themes). Having fitted all the historical facts on the psychohistoriogram, the chart was analyzed, and expressions of the attitudinal positions of persons at specific chronological times were made as literary and emotional themes that would form the organizational framework for writing the pageant, in the language of the people. The labeled themes and trends were then listed on a separate chart. Separate notes were also kept of dynamic group interactions taking place as the group process proceeded. Based on selected themes, trends and dynamic exchanges, designated members were, as part of the process of actualization, assigned tasks that included writing prose and/or poetry, collating historical material, and carrying out research. The major themes culled from the ethnohistorical meetings were:

1. Anecdotes of historical characters and events
2. Mental illness and its causes
3. Socio-political and economic issues
4. Patient and staff communication and morale
5. Patient and staff conflicts
6. Cruel treatment of patients
7. Changing attitudes and practices at Bellevue Hospital
8. Poor working conditions
9. Worker and administration conflict
10. Trade union political struggle.

Anecdotal and folk material thrown up by the group discussion was recorded and entered above and below the timeline on the chart by the analyst. Depending on the clustering of the recorded material, vertical lines were drawn through it and labeled according to the nature of the historical dialectical discussion. These lines were identified as themes and trends, with the interpretation being made by the analyst, and discussed by the group. The insights and themes established the framework of the pageant that was transformed into new creations—poems, prose, songs—that catalyzed empowerment and transformation of the process. As more historical material was recorded, clustering of the incidents soon became apparent. Vertical lines were drawn through the clustered material, establishing significant watershed periods in the collective historical experiences of the group. Each period was named and used as a theme around which dramatic scripts were prepared, illustrating the dynamics of the group. Dramatic pageants with music and poetry were created using these themes and trends, depicting the history of Bellevue Hospital and the struggles of the Jamaican mental health movement.

The role and skill of the psychohistoriographic analyst must be emphasized. Dialectical analysis of group discussion of this nature often generates explosive contradictions within the group, requiring expert and sensitive management. This analysis facilitates insight into contradictory issues and provides new syntheses to contradictions which encourage change and transformation. *The essence of cultural therapy is the dialectical analysis of psychohistoriography* and has been used in a number of different circumstances since the inception of the cultural therapy process. Although psychohistoriography is a stand-alone activity with measurable outcomes, it constitutes only the partial realization of the cultural therapy process. The analysis of historical anecdotes and the dialectical discussion of the paradoxes and contradictions of the group experience lead to the development of thematic watershed lines which in turn provide collective constructs and insights. These thematic constructs and insights have created what is known as the 'psychic centrality' [22]—the psychic essence—of the group.

An example of a theme is represented by reflections concerning the genocidal extermination of the Taino. This led to a conscious thematic statement of the confrontation of the European psychosis by Black people ('We come yah before yu') negating the commonly repeated myth that Caribbean and American history began with the 'discovery' of the

New World by Christopher Columbus. Also shown in Fig. 6.2 is the historical musical development of Jamaican culture and the concrete administrative psychiatric decisions that have influenced psychiatry and attitudes to madness in Jamaica. This was the essential framework for the sociodrama pageant, forming the literary headings, the scene design framework, the actual characters of the drama of history, the musical history, and its sequence. All were taken and woven into *Madnificent Irations*, written in free verse, and reflecting the psychohistorical facts that have influenced the reality of psychiatry in Jamaica today as ascertained by the collective analysis of ethnohistorical representation of the institution. The following pageant themes created the framework of the script:

1. Madness/Badness
2. We come yah before yu/UK 'captures' Jamaica
3. Leave me alone, why yu tek me from mi lan/Maroon repatriation
4. Tek mi home to Africa/Maroon repatriation
5. We want land we want freedom/The fight for freedom
6. Obeah/Anti-Obeah laws – Obeah users mad and bad
7. Release from mental enslavement/Emancipation, asylum built: Lock up the dissidents
8. The messianic visionaries/Custodial care
9. Don't sell us out; freedom for one and for all/UK begins to free the Black man
10. Don't fuck around I man; I want more money/Black Saturday 'Bedlam'
11. Festering in a nest of vipers/Independence under the capitalist system
12. Africa in sight; sociodrama, therapeutic communities/Multinationals, money god.

The script of *Madnificent Irations* (see Appendix) told of a proud tribe of Africans brought across the Atlantic Middle Passage by ruthless Europeans for the explicit purpose of the exploitation of their labor in the plantations and for shameless sexual exploitation of both males and females. The pageant enacted the story of the building of the lunatic asylum in the post-emancipation period for the express purpose of forcible control of rebellious and deviant behaviors of the newly freed slaves and vigorous demands for religious and political freedom. *Madnificent Irations* described the paradox of madness existing in the Jamaican society. The concept of the paradox of the two major opposing forces of the European enslaver and the Africans enslaved in this New World, and the spectrum of potencies ranging from the very good to the very bad, and the very ugly all existing in the same environment. The pageant attempted to describe the European medical model and to distill the nature of the diagnosis of madness that this model portrays. In order to understand the cycle that we have been trapped in, we have to abandon that model and use another archetype that would explain the paradigm of mental illness that captures the lunacy of the European *delusion* which demands the acceptance of *White superiority* on the one hand and moves to negate the demand for *African liberation and negritude* on the other. This paradox can only be resolved by the acceptance of the reality that the entire country must be viewed as a lunatic asylum and that there is a whole spectrum of people in this country who have different degrees of mental illness. *Madnificent Irations* addressed the issue of a structural situation where a small group of people in power are in control of the majority of the population, and drew the audience's attention to the idea of the entire island as a single, giant plantation, effectively a total institution. This plantation in turn morphed into the present-day garrison communities controlled by despotic politicians and ruthless rogue dons, where the politician and the criminal go hand in hand. The pageant described Jamaica in the 1970s, where the whole country was able to confront the reality of the situation at Bellevue Hospital, where the major problem was one of violence and fear of violence. The pageant described the requirement for a mental hospital with the capability to contain and then transform people who were crazy and violent into being sane and relatively unviolent.

In this rehabilitation mode, there are three very clear therapeutic approaches. The first is the *therapeutic community*, where everybody has to sit down every day for an hour and reason with each other, to determine what their productive tasks are for the day and whether they are going to do something positive, such as planting some callaloo. *Madnificent Irations* illustrated the therapeutic need for the mental hospital and the Jamaican community to sit in circles, in groups, to *reason* daily about productivity, activities for daily living, and for a democratic system of managing power and authority. We tried to build into the script of *Madnificent Irations* the therapeutic prescription for the hospital and the country itself. The purpose of the therapeutic community, in which we develop institutional structures to respect one another and to speak civilly to each other, is therefore to address and stop the conflict and violence within ourselves.

The second, *vocational therapy*, ensures that every human being in the country has to be in some form of productive work. It's a huge task, and it's not going to be easy to put a million people to work. The pageant showed that was what we did in Bellevue by putting the entire community to work. In two or three years, we had everybody working, we were growing our own food, having our own plays and entertainment, and of course what we found was that the violence stopped immediately and that people were beginning to live peaceably with each other.

The third prescription, *cultural therapy*, uses the culture of the people to drive the energy of the vocational activity and the psychological decolonization of a people oppressed for four hundred years. We applied it in Bellevue in the period 1977–1982. We taught people to look at their history and how that history impacts on present behavior, and then to use the culture that is innate in them, the music and the drama and the art and everything else, to become productively enhanced, based on that knowledge and that reasoning. The cultural therapy program brought patients who had been warehoused in the asylum for decades to the Garden Theatre daily, first to participate as audience and then to take part in dance and dramatic activities, structured by the psychiatric aides who had been trained in the Edna Manley College of the Visual and Performing Arts.

The entire script was created by the inmates, nurses and aides, with the construction and message of the pageant resonating with the inmates' anguish, pain, and strong desire for freedom. *Madnificent Irations* tells the story through the lens of two narrators (Fig. 6.3) who take on the personae of different historical figures such as Paul Bogle after the Morant Bay Rebellion in 1865. They describe the historical events and transitions both in Jamaica and in the asylum in which they find themselves. The dialogue is between the European enslavers who have brought over the proud tribe of Africans and enslaved them in the New World and specifically in the Caribbean island of Jamaica. Several other minor *madnificent personae*, both men and women, tell the story of their forced migration from Africa and the horrors of plantation life in this new country where the original inhabitants have been genocidally eradicated. The pageant relates the history of Jamaica from the arrival of the British and their cruel exploitative social engineering of the captured Africans from the mid-seventeenth century, and the unequal and abusive

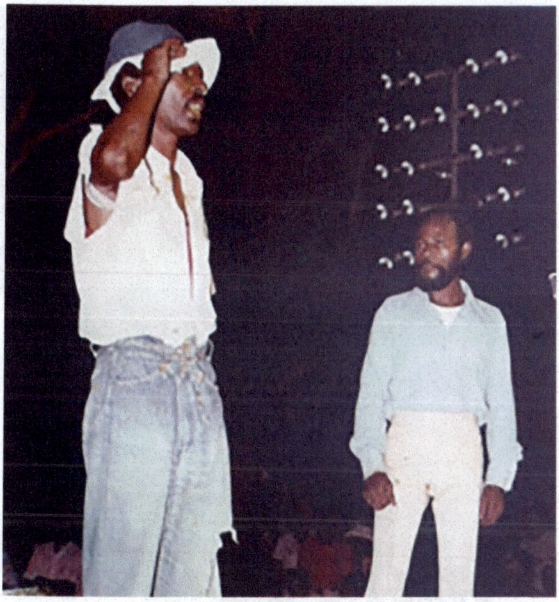

Fig. 6.3 The narrators Madman 1 and Madman 2 lead the discourse in *Madnificent Irations*

sexual and occupational exploitation in the service of the generation of British wealth. The pageant attempts to dramatize the contradictions between the African cultural religious experience that is deemed insanity by the European Christian culture, and the physical and economic hardships endured by the enslaved Africans (Fig. 6.4).

One of the scenes depicts a commonly encountered clinical presentation of mental illness where the patient identifies that they are put upon by Obeah demons who threaten to possess them. For the uninitiated, this can be a very confusing clinical presentation and sometimes quite frightening. This was depicted in the pageant of a patient explaining to his doctor '*She put a duppy pon me Sar!*' A duppy—restless ghost or spirit of the dead—is the word commonly used to describe anything that is connected with the supernatural. Some people make a distinction between the duppy as an evil spirit and other types of spirit, sometimes called 'ancestral', which are good [23, p. 163].

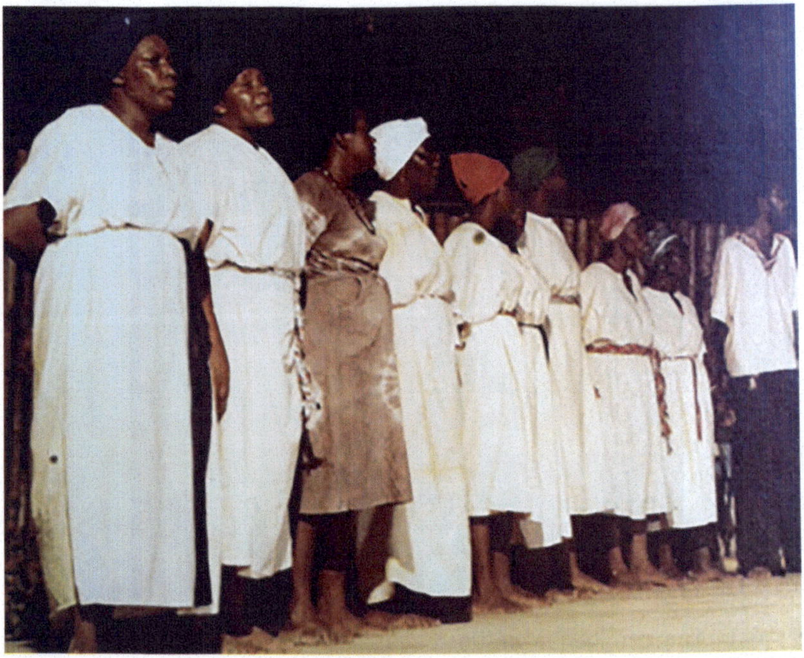

Fig. 6.4 Patients and staff in *Madnificent Irations* portraying 'the proud tribe of Africa' brought to the New World as slaves

Madnificent Irations then re-enacted specific historical watershed events that saw the asylum used as a repository for rebellious ex-slaves and political activists demanding political liberation and large-scale repatriation to Africa. Particular attention was paid to the steely totality of political engineering by the British, who established the colonial governorship, judiciary, military, constabulary, prison and asylum to enforce the absolute authority and hegemony of a small number of Whites over the burgeoning population of Black people in this colony.

The pageant told the story of a particular patient admitted in 1895 named Alexander Bedward, 30 years after the Morant Bay Rebellion which saw hundreds of Black and Creole Jamaicans executed by the British ruling classes. Bedward has become a Jamaican folk hero. He was a revolutionary political leader of the time who had organized a religious revolutionary movement across Jamaica demanding repatriation of Black people to Africa. The colonial government first arrested him and tried him for treason, but when he was found not guilty of the charge they then arrested him under the Lunacy Act and incarcerated him in the asylum. While we were writing and staging *Madnificent Irations*, I found a number of ancient leather-bound ledgers containing the case notes of all the early admissions to the asylum, in the corridor of the administrative building; they had been discarded as garbage by the nursing administrators who were the assigned safekeepers. The documents that I found in one of these ledgers contained numerous newspaper articles about the trial which had found him innocent of the charge of treason and his subsequent admission to the asylum on the grounds of his being of unsound mind. The carefully penned handwritten case notes of his admission and period of incarceration could not corroborate any clinical evidence of lunacy and he eventually had to be released. The notes recorded that Bedward then fled to Costa Rica, where he stayed for the next twenty years. When he returned to Jamaica, the colonial government arrested him again on the grounds of lunacy and incarcerated him in the asylum, where he subsequently died some years later. On this occasion of his readmission, he was accused of having proclaimed to his followers that he was going to ascend to heaven like Elijah in a chariot. This was the evidence of his insanity that was used to legally incarcerate him. Edward White reported that Bedward claimed that he had never intended his talk of flying to heaven to be taken literally [23]. White's account reminded us of tales about men and women blessed with the power of flight that have been a staple of West African folklore for centuries, always with the promise of awakening and liberation.

There are those to this day, White wrote, 'who believe that Bedward's reputation has been deliberately trashed by a concatenation of falsehood and lies'. Devout Bedwardites, White reported, 'dismissed the idea that Bedward was insane as so much white propaganda'. The colonial government that 'Bedward had so thoroughly infuriated and embarrassed' was trying to embellish the Bedward myth and to dilute the revolutionary potency of his message. There is no doubt that this period of Jamaican history, just 30 years after the vicious and bloody Morant Bay Rebellion, had left the colonial leaders in fear of a similar violent uprising, and they used everything in their power to negate and silence that revolutionary threat.

The ledgers contained much information that found its way into *Madnificent Irations.* I rue the day that I did not retrieve all of them for safekeeping before the political repercussions of the cultural therapy struggle resulted in my removal from Bellevue in 1983. These ledgers have been lost to posterity. They were left in the safekeeping of the hospital nursing administration. I have no doubt that they were thrown out, likely in ignorance, by those who denigrated their value. I mentioned this to my colleague Geoffrey Walcott many years later, when we were carrying out an audit of rural hospitals in Jamaica. The matron of one of these hospitals told us that it was hospital policy for patients' dockets to be destroyed after ten years, to make space for the new.

The pageant dramatized a number of 'madman' jokes that have been popular in the Jamaican culture. One tale relates the sale of a pair of shoes by a Bellevue patient to an unsuspecting civilian passer-by who gets duped by the con-artist into buying a pair of shoes with two left feet. This dramatized tale mirrors the theme thread of the pageant of 'Ah who mad, yu or me?' which challenges the audience to distinguish the thin dividing line between sanity and madness.

Another tale relates the story of a patient selling a mule owned by the hospital, reflecting a theme that identified the presence of a number of accomplished con-artists who ended up as fully functional long-stay patients incarcerated in the institution. Terror of the potential violence of lunatics was another thread that ran through the pageant. The scene of a terrified civilian being pursued by a Bellevue lunatic brandishing a machete in his hand, only to be tapped on the shoulder with the childhood playful entreaty '*last lick. Your time to chase me now*,' poked fun at the fear and terror that laypersons have of the propensity of lunatics to violence, not realizing that violent acts of mentally ill people are relatively rare.

One of the early scenes of *Madnificent Irations* dramatized almost verbatim the ravings of a mentally ill young woman whose delusional conflicts were of her father being a White man with long straight hair. This delusion of Brown and Black people psychically considering themselves to be White is a phenomenon reported in 'The Roast Breadfruit Psychosis' (Hickling and Hutchinson) [25]. The pageant dramatized the scene of the delusional madwoman inviting the White colonial doctor who was examining her to sexual engagement and to impregnate her with a White baby. These delusional ideas are very common in Jamaican people and produced a number of uncomfortable and disturbed reactions in audience members who viewed the pageant, including the eminent theatre critic Norman Rae in his *Gleaner* review of *Madnificent Irations* [26]. This is discussed in greater detail in Chapter 7.

Culturing and Cognitive Catalysis

A critical aspect of the psychohistoriographic process in the creation of the script is the use of the oral anecdotes and phrases in the creation of the dramatic activity and the actual scripted lines used. This process has been strongly developed in the process of psychohistoriographic cultural therapy as it has developed in the decades following this first psychohistoriographic pageant and has been called *culturing*. A word, thought, or memory summoned by group cultural reasoning triggers a creative process that we have called *cognitive catalysis*; song lines, poetic lyrics, and dramatic ideas are pursued, honed, and developed jointly with the scriptwriter. The process of *poetic poiesis* involves the creation of neologisms, new songs and lyrics. The ability to create new cultural formations triggers emotional excitement and affective joyfulness that is contagious, enhances consciousness-raising, and inspires individual self-awareness and ability that we have called *capacity building*. In our experience this process has, for all age groups, induced a level of self-confidence and impulse control that has proved to be therapeutic and enduring.

The Processes Involved in Patient Transformation

The question is, what was the essence of this transformation process in terms of the patients? What was the process, what was driving it, what was the effect? Was there long-term study of its effectiveness? In a study published in 1989, the progress of a group of patients who were involved in the cultural therapy process was compared against that of the control group, who were not. The factors used to measure improvement included reduced levels of medication and increased involvement in group activities [27]. The process was able to unlock the social and psychological problems affecting Black people in post-slave societies that have come about as a result of slavery. It is related to 'smadification' ('smady' meaning 'somebody' in Jamaican dialect), the process of acquiring resiliency and personhood [28].

Ethnohistoriography, employing a variety of methodologies, involves gathering people together in a large group to discuss their own ethnohistorical identity, based on their own anecdotal histories. The historiography that Becker and Goveia described is a technique that uses books and written material as the basis of the dialectical understanding of history. In Jamaica, we have a paucity of books, so in our understanding of our historiography we have to use the books in people's heads. Psychohistoriography is a technique whereby the members of an ethnic group, whether it be small or large, gather to discuss their anecdotes, their thoughts, their memories, their history, things that they know, and then put this knowledge into an organized dialectical framework, a dialectical sequence. Psychohistoriography has created a technique where we can record these anecdotes that people have as events in their memories and put them into a chronological timeline and into a dialectical analytical framework so that we can understand how the perspectives of truth or untruth color perceptions. To give an example, Christopher Columbus, as seen by Europeans, was an explorer and a discoverer, but to us he was an invader, a thief and a murderer. The dialectical antipodes of these perceptions shape the process of reality formation; psychohistoriography forces people to look at the dialectical perceptions of different recorded facts of history in their own lives and catalyzes the confrontation of myth and the process of insight.

An Obeah man is much closer to this process than any European psychotherapist. We are now beginning to examine and to teach this process at the University of the West Indies; as we begin to understand the various elements, we have increasingly found ourselves amazed at what we are discovering. The major aspect of this particular process is that it deals with the here and now and the realities of people's lives and not with any kind of esoteric abstract understanding of the unconscious mind and the business of unconscious drives and other similar kinds of motivation. The process moves us in exactly the opposite direction from the European context, that did not come out of our experience, but which emerged from the culture of nineteenth-century Vienna. That's the European perception and it has not worked particularly well for them, so why should we believe that it would work for us? We are looking at psychotherapy from the point of view of brain processes and how the brain works, and how people in a cultural activity area work; and then translate it both as individual and collective types of therapies. The psychohistoriographic technique has become the basic element of the cultural therapy process that has been used in subsequent projects in various locations across the world in the forty years following the creation of *Madnificent Irations*. The cultural therapy process at Bellevue Hospital produced three additional sociodramas, *Visionated Penetrations* (1979), *Madaptations* (1980), and *Irations Explosion* (1981), which were performed island-wide to audiences of thousands.

Stage 3: Staging and Production

The Music of Madnificent Irations

Creation of the script drew heavily on the folk songs that are extremely popular in the Jamaican folkloric culture, which in turn triggered great excitement in the creation of dances that accompanied these songs. 'In her book *Forty Folk Songs of Jamaica*, Olive Lewin classifies the songs into 11 groups: Bruckins, Jankunnu, Kumina, Maroon, Mento, Nagos, Rasta (Rastafarian), Revival, (Set-Up; Gerreh), Tambo, and Worksongs. Of these, Mento is by far the most common. However, much of Mento is of relatively recent origin and should be classified as popular music rather than folk' (https://www.wikiwand.com/en/Jamaican_folk music and [29]). Revivalism began in Jamaica between 1860 and 1861 as part of a religious movement called the Great Revival. It is a combination of elements drawn from African beliefs and Christianity and has several forms, the two major forms being Revival Zion and Pocomania. Less widely diffused and in parallel is the religious form called Myalism, the strongest neo-African cult in Jamaica, which stems from an ancient West African Ashanti ancestor possession cult and incorporates an African worldview in terms of its understanding of nature, deity, and human relationships. Myalism is related to Pocomania, which represents the union of Myalism and Protestant Christianity in Jamaica [30].

The songs used in *Madnificent Irations* emerged from the players themselves. Many of the patients and workers involved in the cultural therapy movement were steeped in Jamaican religious practices and knew 'by ear' the music of their ancestors. The songs used in the pageant came mainly from Revival, Pocomania, or Baptist Revival sources. As the script emerged, specific songs were suggested by the performers to characterize the scene being enacted and often the lyrics were modified to correspond with the emerging script. Some of the songs were collective creations of the performers or the Irations Band. As audio-visual recordings of the performances were not made, the actual music of the songs remains only in the memories of some of the remaining participants. Each song has been listed, and a summary of its origin will be attempted.

Dread Lion. The concept of 'Dread Lion' was very popular in the Jamaican parlance and was immortalized by Lee 'Scratch' Perry (Rainford Hugh Perry) and his band The Upsetters in the song of the same title on the 1976 album *Super Ape*. Scratch Perry is a Jamaican music producer and singer noted for his innovative studio techniques and production style [31]. 'Dread Lion' was proposed by the lead actor in *Madnificent Irations* to replace 'madman' in the local lexicon.

'Du Muriah Mama,' 'Fire, Fire, Fire, Fire Fall on Me,' and 'When My Pilot Come' are well-known Pentecostal Revival songs of uplift. 'Modder de Grave Stone Gotta Move,' 'John Saw Them Coming,' and 'Jah Jah Go Before Us' are inspirational prophetic songs from the Pocomania genre that fit right into the *Madnificent Irations* history of the struggle of Africans enslaved in the New World (Fig. 6.5).

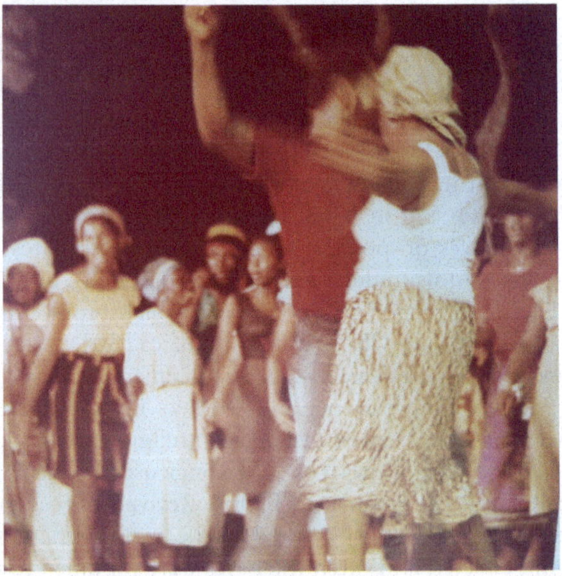

Fig. 6.5 Folkloric song and dance *Cut Muno*

Ten Pound Ten Fe Got Cut Muno: (Cut Muno: A man seeking sex). The origin of this song is unclear, but it is likely that it arose in the early Mento period, and is the refrain of a man seeking sex for money and reflected the state of sexual deprivation encountered in the asylum.

Ten poun ten fe go cut muno
wai oh, wai oh
Ten poun ten fe go cut muno
wai oh, wai oh
Big muno small muno fat muno
wai oh, cut muno

Gimmie House, Gimmie Clothes, Gimmie Food Fe Eat was a refrain created by the performers and appears on more than one occasion in the pageant, reflecting periods of hunger and destitution experienced by the Jamaican people as part of our history.

Jane and Louisa is a ring play game song originating in the Mento genre made popular by Jamaican poet and entertainer Louise Bennett in the early 1950s.

Sly Mongoose: The music of the folk songs such as 'Sly Mongoose' disguised a message of resistance and rebellion of Bedwardism of the Jamaican people against the British colonizer [32].

Sly mongoose yuh name gone abroad,
mongoose go ina Bedward kitchen,
tek out one of him righteous chicken,
put it ina him waistcoat pocket, sly mongoose.

The mongoose was the cultural designation of the White butcher (the colonial government) who had invaded Bedward's kitchen in order to steal his 'righteous chicken' (the message of his business) in order to prevent him from carrying out his revolutionary activity. When he was first arrested, the charge of treasonous or rebellious activity could not be substantiated and he was incarcerated instead in the asylum. The ancient case records that we had stumbled on were the actual clinical records of the British doctors who were unable to find evidence of clinical psychopathology in Bedward. This rich cultural history was incorporated in *Madnificent Irations* as we crafted the history of madness in Jamaica in this cultural performance.

Dip dem Bedward: This Jamaican folk song gives brief descriptions of the many persons, from all over Jamaica, who came to the healing services conducted by the shepherd (Bedward) of a very large Revival church between the 1890s and the early twentieth century.

Chorus:
Oh!
Dip dem Bedward, dip dem
Dip dem in di healing stream,
Dip dem deep, but not too deep;
Dip dem fi cure bad feeling.

Verse 1:
Some come from the east
Like a big leggo beast,
Fi guh dip inna di healing stream.
Some come from the west
Like a perfect pest,
Fi guh dip inna di healing stream.

Verse 2:
Some come from the north
Wid dem face full a wart,
Fi guh dip inna di healing stream.
Some come from the south
Wid dem big yabba mouth,
Fi guh dip inna di healing stream.

A *leggo beast* is someone that is under no control; it also is a definition of a loose woman [32]. A *yabba* is an earthenware bowl of West African origin. In this context, it is an uncomplimentary aspersion on big thick negro lips [33]. The healing stream was the Hope River in August Town, St. Andrew, where Bedward had his church and performed ritual baptism. Bedward was a household name in Jamaica, and membership of his church grew prodigiously, with branches all over Jamaica and disciples in Cuba, Panama, and Costa Rica. His power and influence profoundly disturbed the leaders of Jamaican society and colonial authorities, as he always attributed deprivation and oppression of the masses to White enslavers and colonialists. He frequently mentioned the Morant Bay Rebellion of 1865, identifying with the rebels' cause. He was arrested and convicted of being a lunatic in 1921 and died in the asylum on November 8, 1930.

Feel Sey I Want to be Free was a song created by the Irations Band to fill the space in the pageant that reflected the deep-seated feeling for freedom felt by the inmates of the hospital and the people of Jamaica.

Step by Step: Seated in a circle, the Bellevue Cultural Therapy Team created the collective song 'Step by Step' in response to the creative search for a fitting finale to the sociodrama. Five drummers provided the Rastafarian rhythmic background and each line was forged out of the participative contributions of the group, led by the cultural therapist who guided the lyrical and musical content. Lyrics and music were written down and recorded by one of the nurses of the group.

Gimmie Back Me Shilling Wid de Lion Pon It: In the pre-independence period, the currency of exchange was sterling (i.e. pounds, shillings and pence), a very stable currency. A Jamaican coin, the penny ha'penny (or quartile, known colloquially as a 'quattie') resembled a tiny version of the shilling. The Jamaican saying 'quattie show the shape (resembles exactly in diminutive form) of the shilling' thus draws an inference of resemblance in any social circumstance. A coin central to the life of the working poor disappeared following a devaluation, causing increased hardship. This song emerged as a protest song against currency devaluation and oppression and fitted perfectly into the pageant analysis and scripting.

Oh de Woman ina Kitchen She a Grumble Sey She Want Go: A Mento song providing a glimpse of early twentieth-century Jamaican working-class life.

Ah Penny Wheel Oh a Penny Wheel: This Mento song, also a product of the early twentieth century, reflects the growth of prostitution in the cities during a period of great economic hardship. The 'penny wheel' was the cheapest form of 'purchased' sex. The line *'wey mek yu push yu cushy gi mi penny wheel'* expressed a sentiment of rebuke and shame. 'Cushy' is the Jamaican dialectical word for vagina [33].

Eastern Standard Time: Jamaican trombonist Don Drummond (*aka* Don Cosmic, *aka* Malungu) died at Bellevue in 1969. Long regarded as one of the world's foremost trombone players, he was one of the architects of ska, which emerged in the early 1960s [34]. His musical genius generated more than 500 songs and ska remains the only genre of music in which the trombone provides the lead with the trumpet and saxophone providing the secondary harmonies. Drummond's love affair with rhumba dancer Anita 'Margarita' Mahfood ended on 31 December, 1965, with her fatal stabbing in Kingston. He was found guilty of her murder by reason of insanity in 1967. *Eastern Standard Time* was one of his most important creations in the expression of explosive cultural creativity fuelling Jamaica's postcolonial search for psychological and economic freedom from the ravages of four hundred years of British slavery and colonial exploitation [34]. This piece found a fitting place in the script of *Madnificent Irations*, locating a starring performing role for Eleazor 'Trummie' Beckford, featured trombonist of the Irations Band, and a cell-mate of Don Drummond in the mid-1960s.

Bibliography

1. Hickling FW (1985) Poem "Westminster System" (Unpublished).
2. Hickling FW (2004) *From Explanitations and Madnificent Irations to de Culcha Clash*: Popular Theatre as Psychotherapy. *Interventions: International Journal of Post-Colonial Studies, 6*(1), 45–66.
3. Kidd R (1980) People's Theatre, Conscientization and Struggle. *Media Development, 27*(3), 10–14.
4. Freire P (1972) *Pedagogy of the Oppressed.* Harmondsworth: Penguin Books.
5. Freire P (1977) *Pedagogy in Process: The Letters to Guinea Bissau.* Trans CSJ Hunter. New York: Seabury.
6. Hamilton B (1988) Marcus Garvey and Cultural Development in Jamaica. In R Lewis, P Bryan (Eds.), *Garvey: His Work and Impact.* Kingston: Institute of Social and Economic Research & Department of Extra-Mural Studies, University of the West Indies, pp. 87–111.
7. Bennett W, Bennett H (2011) *The Jamaican Theatre: Highlights of the Performing Arts in the Twentieth Century.* Kingston: University of the West Indies Press.
8. Hickling FW (2005) Catalyzing Creativity. In F Hickling, E Sorel (Eds.), *Images of Psychiatry, The Caribbean.* Kingston: Department of Community Health and Psychiatry, University of the West Indies, Mona Campus.
9. Hickling FW, Griffith EEH (1994) Clinical Perspectives on the Rastafari Movement. *Hospital and Community Psychiatry, 45*(1), 49–53.
10. Hickling FW (2007). *Psychohistoriography: A Post-colonial Psychoanalytic and Psychotherapeutic Model.* Kingston: CARIMENSA, University of the West Indies.
11. Hickling FW (1989) Sociodrama in the Rehabilitation of Chronic Mental Illness. *Hospital and Community Psychiatry, 40*, 402–406.
12. Hickling FW (2004) Popular Theatre as Psychotherapy. *Interventions: International Journal of Post-Colonial Studies, 6*(1), 45 56.
13. Goveia EV (1956) *A Study on the Historiography of the British West Indies to the End of the Nineteenth Century.* Mexico: Instituto Panamericano de Geografia.

14. Becker C (1938) What Is Historiography? *American Historical Review, 44*, 1–28.
15. Jaspers K (1923) *Allgemeine Pathologie*. Berlin: Springer Verlag; (1963) *General Psychopathology* (Translated from the German by J Hoenig, MW Hamilton). Manchester: Manchester University Press, pp. 712–713.
16. Hickling FW (2007) The Components of Psychohistoriographic Cultural Therapy (Chapter 4). In FW Hickling, *Psychohistoriography: A Post-colonial Psychoanalytic and Psychotherapeutic Model.* Kingston: CARIMENSA, University of the West Indies.
17. Brodber E (1983) Oral Sources and the Creation of a Social History of the Caribbean. *Jamaica Journal, 16*(4), 2–11.
18. Mbiti JS (1969) *African Religions and Philosophy.* London: Heinemann, pp. 16–17.
19. Mills C (1997) *The Racial Contract.* Ithaca and London: Cornell University Press.
20. Norman G (1975) Aspects of the Political Economy of Race in the Caribbean. *Working Paper Series, No 7*, Mona ISER.
21. Rouse R (1860) *New Light on Dark Deeds; Being Jottings from the Diary of Richard Rouse, Late Warden of the Lunatic Asylum of Kingston. Edited by his son.* Kingston: Hall and Myers.
22. Hickling FW, Guzder J, Robertson-Hickling H, Snow S, Kirmayer LJ (2010) Psychic Centrality: Reflections on Two Psychohistoriographic Workshops in Montreal. *Transcultural Psychiatry, 47*, 136.
23. White E (2016) Rise Up: Alexander Bedward's Mythical Powers of Flight. *The Paris Review,* October 5, https://www.theparisreview.org/blog/2016/10/05/rise-up/.
24. Senior O (2003) *Encyclopaedia of the Jamaican Heritage.* St. Andrew, Jamaica: Twin Guinep.
25. Hickling FW, Hutchinson G (1999) The Roast Breadfruit Psychosis: Disturbed Racial Identification in African Caribbeans. *Psychiatric Bulletin, 23*, 132–134.
26. Rae N (1978) 'A Line from the Tower of Babble: Madnificent Irations at the Bellevue Garden Theatre'. *Gleaner*, September 10.
27. Hickling FW (1989) Sociodrama in the Rehabilitation of Chronic Mentally Ill Patients. *Hospital and Community Psychiatry, 40*, 402–406.
28. Scott D, Nettleford, RM (2006) "To Be Liberated from the Obscurity of Themselves": An Interview with Rex Nettleford. *Small Axe, 10*(2), 97–246.
29. Lewin O (1973) *Forty Folk Songs of Jamaica. Collected and transcribed by Olive Lewin.* Washington: General Secretariat of the Organization of American States
30. Scott S (2018) The Rise of Revivalism in Jamaica. *Jamaica Observer Sunday,* January 21.

31. Strong MC (2000) *The Great Rock Discography* (5th ed.). Edinburgh: Mojo Books, pp. 738–741.
32. Hickling FW, Hutchinson G (2012) Madness as Social Defiance in African Caribbean Youth: Evidence from the Dancehall. *Wadabagei: A Journal of the Caribbean and Its Diasporas, 13*(3), 3–25.
33. Cassidy FG, LePage RB (1980) *Dictionary of Jamaican English* (2nd ed.). Kingston: University of the West Indies Press.
34. Augustyn H (2013) *Don Drummond: The Genius and Tragedy of the World's Greatest Trombonist.* Jefferson, NC: McFarland Publishers.

CHAPTER 7

The Impact of *Madnificent Irations*

Let us waken from de slumber
Of de anaesthetic gas
Which has kept us in de ghettos
Of de men's mental morass. [1]

Stages 4 and 5: Performance and Evaluation

Madnificent Irations played for 27 performances at the Bellevue Garden Theatre and subsequently toured the island. It was seen by over 25,000 people. There was an outpouring of support for the pageant in the local media. In the first year, the performance received two theatrical newspaper reviews, and was the subject of eleven newspaper reports and four television commentaries. The news media had difficulty in deciding how to report on the performance. In some articles the pageant was described as a social/historical event, while in others, written by professional theatre reviewers, it was treated as a bona fide theatrical production. A product of the cultural therapy process, *Madnificent Irations* was the first of four sociodramas performed at Bellevue Hospital between 1978 and 1982. A media representation analysis comparing all newspaper articles about reports on mental health issues between 1974 and 1985 showed that the cultural therapy process triggered a 500% increase (14 reports in 1975 and 85 reports in 1981) in newspaper articles about mental health (Fig. 7.1).

Verena Reckord, a well-known theatre reviewer, described *Madnificent Irations* as 'a living indication of the tremendous results that

F. W. Hickling, *Decolonization of Psychiatry in Jamaica*,
https://doi.org/10.1007/978-3-030-48489-7_7

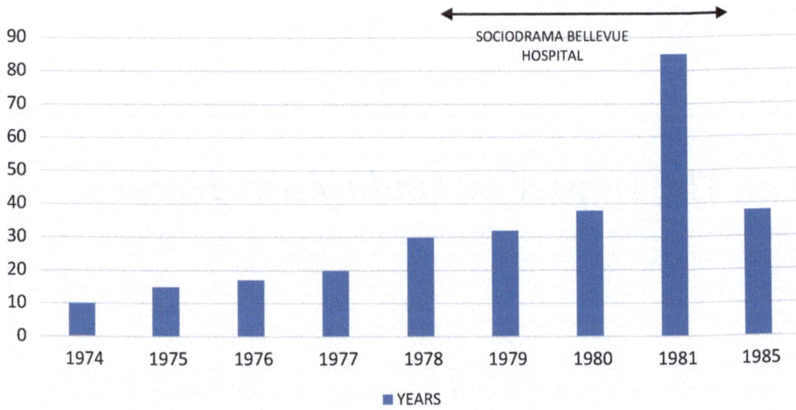

Fig. 7.1 Newspaper responses to sociodrama performances at Bellevue Hospital

can come from concerted community endeavour...it was not only produced by the Bellevue community, but that group also built, by hand—the staff and patients together—the very formidable, but attractive, bamboo garden theatre'. She continued: 'The Bellevue Garden Theatre, as it is called, is well laid out, with a spacious tiered brick floor, a vast circular stage, framed by large lignum vitae trees...this historical pageant—in song, dance, and drama—shows that the original concept of the Bellevue Hospital as a mere "madhouse" is no longer true' [2] (Fig. 7.2). Reckord reported that the script described Blacks who tried to move out of the colonial mold and who insisted on preserving their own African culture were called crazy for doing so. In those days, according to the script, the 'madhouse' and the 'penitentiary' were the colonial rulers' answer to keeping the Blacks in check. One jail in question, built the same year as the madhouse, was that veritable monument to colonial oppressive programs—the General Penitentiary on Tower Street. This kind of information and more came to the audience, via a large beautifully controlled cast of patients and staff of Bellevue Hospital.

She went on to describe the pageant as a large if somewhat loose but complex weave of historical events from 1862 till the present day. The basic threads represented the prevailing inhumane conditions (for staff and patients) at the hospital, and the painfully slow stages of improvement over the years. She considered that the play was somewhat

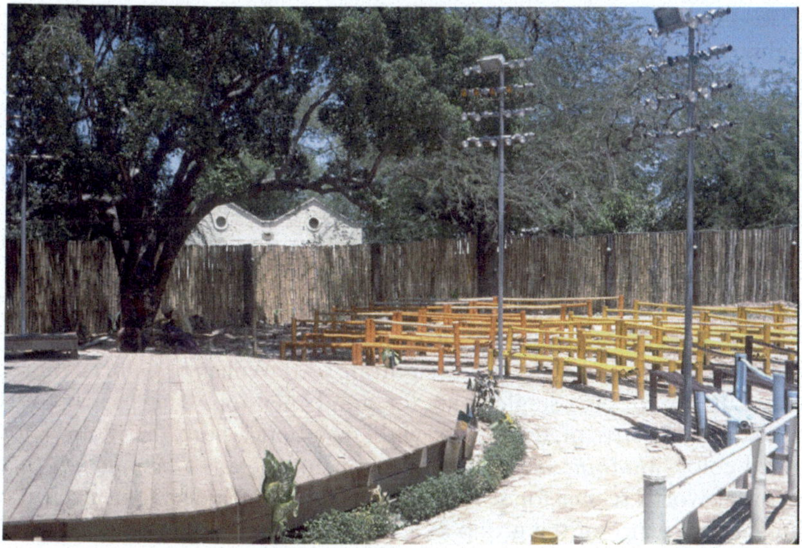

Fig. 7.2 Bellevue Garden Theatre stage

opinionated, but that there was a great deal of logic in the weaving of other historical 'data.' The pattern included the behavior of developed and developing countries over the years and the cause and effect of events, at the domestic and regional levels, at parochial and universal levels. She reported that quite a bit of attention was focused on the cultural history of Jamaica, as reflected in folk songs and dances which were economically applied in the progression of the pageant. The overriding message throughout was that 'we should go into our "headcups", that is, use our own minds to think-out our problems and find our own solutions, because that is possible with the right kind of thinking'. Also in the threads of *Madnificent Irations* was the message that the fight for Black and Third World freedom continued. In terms of living standards and other sociopolitical conditions, this has only just begun, and needs to be intensified. The 'colorful and at times funny production' was also, she felt, very realistic, bringing many social ills into sharp focus, simultaneously reflecting a view of the day-to-day problems and happenings outside of Bellevue. Reckord opined that the script could benefit from cutting, but that it did not use social commentaries just for laughs, but to underscore valid serious comment.

Reckord also noted that the pageant underscored the potentially highly therapeutic nature of theatrical experience. She considered that with everyone acting so well and working together as a team, on and off stage, it was difficult for the audience to tell patients from staff, thus reflecting on the thin line between madness and sanity. All things considered, she said, the players did justice to their roles and that it was difficult to single out any of the performers for individual commendation.

That said, Reckord made specific mention of Lockhart Hines, who played Madman and Narrator. She opined that he was a fine showman, with a voice and movement qualities that were just right for the part. Hines was a very good storyteller and actor who held the audience's attention at all times. Denise Creighton, Cliff Williams, Gilbert Binns, and others were also singled out for good mention. The pageant was backed by a corps of drummers with trombone, flute, harmonica for added color. *Madnificent Irations*, she concluded, was a production that was well worth seeing for several reasons and concluded that given the limited experience of the group as a whole the production ranged highly in competence, entertainment value, interest and was worthy of support.

The *Daily Gleaner* report of Tuesday 5 September 1978 included two photographs of the audience at the performance and the pageant, the latter featuring Lockhart Hines as Madman [3]. In a commentary by Nana, a number of the issues raised by the other *Daily News* reporters were also captured; many of the themes uncovered by the psychohistoriographic analysis were clearly identified [4]. Nana described *Madnificent Irations* as an interesting experiment in which patients and staff of the Bellevue Hospital staged a pageant telling about themselves and their lives in an institution that was feared by many outside its walls. Nana related that:

> It was fascinating to watch the performance of *Madnificent Irations*. It was equally fascinating to watch the audience reaction. To hear people trying to make out who was patient and who was staff. The play could be seen as a method of treatment. Not just for those defined as being 'mad,' but also for those who sat and watched. It demanded that we look at the way we understand mental illness, and our treatment of the mentally ill. Bellevue Hospital was built, shortly after emancipation, at about the same time as the General Penitentiary (GP), a few yards down the road, and was intended to perform much the same function as the prison. Those in the GP were deemed criminals by society and called 'bad,' while those in

Bellevue were called 'mad.' Both institutions could be viewed as ways colonial rulers found to contain the newly freed Black population. It has taken over one hundred years for both of them to move away from being massive prisons, and to start dealing with rehabilitating those who do not live up to the community's standards of behavior.

Nana opined that most of us do not realize that a person is mentally ill until their behavior becomes obviously inappropriate and that we feel that all mentally ill persons are violent, thus ignoring the signposts to their eventual outburst. Nana suggested that our lack of understanding about the process of mental illness contributed to our fear of those we call mad and that we do not recognize how much we contribute individually and collectively to an individual's mental health. The majority of patients at Bellevue were very poor. She provided an example of a woman, a former patient, who came requesting readmission. Her house had burned to the ground and she had nowhere to go except Bellevue. Another example concerned a young man admitted with a form of psychosis. Although he recovered after a few days of treatment, the nurses knew that they would see him again in a few weeks as he was unemployed, his family had thrown him out, and he had nothing to do but sit on the corner and worry on an empty stomach.

Nana described the pageant as a most public aspect of efforts that were being made to reorganize the Bellevue Hospital, with patients now being involved in a poultry project and in the area of craft development. The Garden Theatre had been built by patients and staff and these vocational activities were aimed at helping mentally ill persons become useful members of society. Nana's media commentary was a valuable contribution to health education, emphasizing the ways in which the community can accept persons discharged from the hospital. The pageant brought to light the ways in which therapeutic events for the mentally ill in Jamaica have affected the patients and staff of the hospital and the community audience. The pageant, Nana suggested, demanded that we do not reject those we call mad, and lock them away in a 'madhouse'; it made us aware that there is often very little difference between sanity and madness; that 'dem mad people' were very much a part of us and a product of our society.

The degree of sophistication attained by the Bellevue Players soon began to create a major impression in Jamaica. The news media played a very important role in disseminating these insights about decolonization to the wider community. In another *Jamaica Gleaner* commentary, seasoned newspaper reviewer and drama critic Harry Milner reviewed the performance of *Irations Explosion* that he witnessed at Kingston's Little Theatre in September 1982 [5]:

> Having missed previous theatrical performances, or sociodramas as director Fred Hickling prefers to call them, I was really astonished at the standard of the production at the Little Theatre last Tuesday night. Perhaps I should not have been so surprised, for after all, Fred Hickling has had heavy connections with the NDTC over the years and they are one of the few companies who have been regularly capable of adjusting to the difficulties of that theatre where so many groups have come to grief. Moreover, the director has had 30 members of his staff trained to a degree at the Jamaica school of drama. Having in the past year seen some particularly trashy efforts by professional and semiprofessional groups, it was most refreshing to see theatre of this standard, where one might have been expected to have made allowances. And although, naturally the show was far from sophisticated and sometimes lacked polish, very few allowances except for occasional forgetting of lines had to be made at all. What indeed was so enjoyable was the dialect, which was clearly natural to most of the staff, was happily free of the gabbling and shouting which leads to much unintelligibility even in the *panto* [the local annual pantomime] these days, and heard even from experienced actors and actresses becomes, I'm assured, unintelligibility even to many born Jamaicans…

This professional theatre critic for the *Gleaner* did not hold back in his criticism of the theatrical and scripting weaknesses, but judged the performance on the basis of its theatrical merit:

> …the music, singing, and dancing was another matter. To my mind a great deal of the pop singing was far more enjoyable than much of the reggae that had to be endured by alleged professionals. The music was not confined to reggae but included revival, ska, mento and early jazz. The band I found especially interesting, for apart from the skilled modern playing of the guitar there was some very spontaneous jazz playing by trombone and sax. Eleazor Beckford on trombone had the same approach in playing the instrument in the old rugged slide method, that lovers of such early jazz players such as Miff Mole and the Dixieland and New Orleans style, treasure. What was particularly well handled in the show was the chorus dancing and movement which was disciplined as well as enthusiastic. The script was possibly the weakest element but clearly it had to be simple and except for the propaganda, the end was never boring…

But not all of the newspaper articles that appeared following the production of *Madnificent Irations* in 1978 were positive or congratulatory. The article by leading Jamaican theatre newspaper critic Norman Rae was distinctly caustic and condemnatory. He wrote [6]:

> **The MADNIFICENCE** began at the entrance to Bellevue Hospital where I asked the way to the new Garden Theatre. The obliging gentleman stuck out his right hand. As he was facing me, I duly turned left and set out on an unscheduled after-dark tour of the grounds. There was no sign of lights, roads seemed to stretch into the blackness, from time to time bodies stirred in the undergrowth – not necessarily patients but quite likely from the world beyond the ripped zinc fences and the yards on the eastern boundaries. No doubt unconsciously influenced by unenlightened fear of madmen but certainly consciously by prudence when one hesitates to wander in lonely woodland, I thought I might have to forgo participation in *Madnificent Irations*, turned the car around and headed back to the gateway. The obliging gentleman asked whether I had found what I wanted. I hadn't. NO, no, said he, it's this way, pointing with the same right hand. As we were facing in exactly opposite directions from when we first met, he turned out a more reliable guide this time. The Garden Theatre is to the right when you come through the main entrance.
>
> The auditorium, which I am told was built by patients and staff, has a pleasing atmosphere. The twelve-sided, low, wooden stage, a platform really, squats under lignum vitae trees. Bricks pave the courtyard attractively, and lacquered bamboo gleams as the surrounding fence. On the way in, booths display craftwork, and there is ample parking space in the grounds.
>
> For reasons already indicated, the performance was already underway when I got seated. I can't therefore comment on the opening statements which may have explained why a presentation whose PR people had billed as a pageant dealing with the history of the treatment of mental illness in Jamaica, or alternatively as a history of Bellevue hospital, turned out minimally that, perhaps half-a-dozen facts through the whole three hour plus evening, and principally an exposition of Dread consciousness. That such consciousness is based on sheer illiteracy, resentment and absence of self-reliance or the desire to organize the management of one's own destiny, may well be the principal impression that comes through. Obviously this was hardly intended. And the resolution seemed to lie in the chalice services and the locksmen at the end (with careful explanation that the real wisdom weed was not in use). Indeed, the auditorium and the concept of the proceedings with its forty-odd cast on stage plus musicians shay-shaying between occasional skits and continuous polemic, might have lent itself to audience participation to ease the lengthy passage of time.

Give the audience its due, it loved the madmen jokes (generally based on the 'who is mad, you or me?' line) for had we not come as at a zoo to gape at the crazy folk? – and the ladies who threw up their skirts and flaunted their hot pants; it roared at the r…s and the f…s …, recovered boisterously for the munos, and sometimes approved the hatred of Baldhead (the white man) which is *Madnificent Irations'* theme. Flipping through the centuries' history well-nigh according to API [Jamaica Government Agency for Public Information] … for the most part we were in National Heroes country (to digress for a moment, isn't it sad that with the volume of historical research in the West Indies at academic level so little has been communicated popularly; our awareness limits monotonously to the gentlemen that decorate our dollar bills). Irations begins with the slave ships. Its view on the abolition of slavery, Baldhead said "free dem but still downpress dem; given half a chance, he would do it (slavery) all over again". It don't change, says Mad I. Baldhead strip I and I of our culture. Later on "Baldhead own all the lan, strip from I an I father han" (as the Arawak may have said to the Spaniard!). Among the Black man's attributes (not many of which are listed) we learn, is the ability to whistle so only a dog hears; working out a calendar based on the four week cycle of the moon, and the possession of psychic powers. This clearly led to the outlawing of Obeah. In any case, Baldhead said there is no such thing as a mad slave. It's no more than pocomania. Ah Babylon; is just Babylon, Rasta!

Bellevue was built at the same time as the prison (by dem calendar) Mad I tells us in one rare moment of fact. Then it goes on to say that this was because the way to control the naaga, Baldie reckoned, was to build a prison and a madhouse. It is not easy to follow the leap from this to Paul Bogle leading his men to Morant Bay (our tribe is a brave tribe) except it offers an opportunity once again to suggest Baldie's hypocrisy in recalling that …clat Governor Eyre. "Come on home and have a rest; we'll give you a manor" (or that's what it sounded like). Did Eyre not have some more serious disciplinary problems to face on his return to England? But Mad I approaches facts quite cavalierly. It has interesting turns, not only of phrase (the ghetto of the canefield), the attribution of guilt; all the disease, the white man disease dida lick down de yout dem. Hero worship the immortal Che, we expect, and that Fidel freed Cuba from backra massa; but hardly the Coral Gardens incident as a blow in the struggle for freedom, but also of conviction. Bedward's celestial aerodynamics were a Baldhead fabrication in order to lock him away in the asylum. But then the white race is the cruellest and most sadistic of all races in mankind. "Let I go" says Mad I, apparently unaware of two important points – we have been independent for 16 years now, and Baldhead doesn't care too much what happens to us.

> I wish one could feel that Mad I is designed as therapy, that it might help by allowing patients to act out their frustrations publicly and so exorcise some of the demons, but I understand that participants are mainly Psychiatric Aides with just about ten percent patient participation. Alternatively that it was demonstrating stock attitudes to insanity which need to be changed, e.g. when it tells us that the hospital was virtually a prison at one time which no one should escape. It says this was again a white/black thing. Surely a lot of mental institutions throughout the world had/have the same lock up view. In any case, Mad I is silent on what needs to be done. Let I go? Alternatively, that in a subtle way, Mad I's script writer and director S.M.O. Freddie Hickling was saying that "madness' here springs from the resentment of black against white (even in sex matters – the mad girl who says that my father has long, pretty hair. I am a princess ... come f... me nuh?) but that is too great a simplification and what IS to be done about it; the chalice; Dreams of Mother Africa? Let I go? The case history is written up; is there no cure?...

Rae's sarcasm, anger, and slamming condemnation of the pageant of the mental hospital's astounding achievement was palpable and, in my view, reflected openly the fear and terror experienced by this 'sophisticated' Oxonian Jamaica Scholar and contemporary social leader. From when I was a schoolboy growing up in urban Kingston, Jamaica, I have been aware of the fear and terror that Jamaican people have about mental illness and about Bellevue Hospital. To most people, Bellevue, mental illness and terror were synonymous and all roads for the mentally ill led there. While things have changed drastically in terms of the contemporary management of mental illness, the knee-jerk reaction remains, even though today 90% of patients are never admitted to the hospital. From childhood, there have been a plethora of 'madman' jokes about Bellevue, and outrageous myths about the practice of committal to the hospital of the mentally ill. It was a strongly held myth in my childhood that people were paid thirty shillings or a tin of cocoa for taking a mentally ill person to Bellevue. All in all, the concept of the hospital was synonymous with fear and terror. So, for most Jamaicans in 1978, the thought of attending a pageant in the grounds of the hospital would have been seen as the epitome of madness and the anxiety and discomfort expressed by Rae at the beginning of the article would have elicited the sympathy of readers who could identify with the emotions that he expressed when he wrote that he was '*...unconsciously influenced by unenlightened fear of madmen...*' as he drove blindly and helplessly around the grounds of the hospital in the pitch blackness of the Jamaican night.

Rae's attempt to belittle the effect of the process by suggesting that the majority of the players were nursing aides was untrue and distasteful. In fact, the proportion of patient performers involved in productions mounted during the sociodrama period of cultural therapy between 1977 and 1983 ranged between 30% and 60%. His attempt to belittle the role of nursing aides in helping to guide and assist seriously mentally ill people to attain health and achievement was therefore unworthy. Also, Rae's historical comprehension of the fate of the British Governor Eyre, although being technically correct, only portrayed one side—the Anglophile side—of the truth. A public outcry in England did indeed lead to the appointment of a Royal Commission of Inquiry in 1865 into the events on the island. However, this vindicated and exonerated Eyre, commending him for his skill, promptitude, and vigor in suppressing the rebellion. In gently slapping Eyre on the wrist for his murderous and excessively barbaric acts, the Commission found that martial law had been continued too long and that the punishments given had been excessive. On the other hand, attempts were made to bring Eyre to trial for murder. John Stuart Mill and other English liberals organized the Jamaica Committee, which demanded Eyre's prosecution. The Jamaica Committee only succeeded in charging Eyre with a list of misdemeanors. In 1868 he was found not guilty but was then harassed by a series of civil suits. In 1872, Parliament voted Eyre £4133 to defray the costs of these prosecutions, and he was given a pension as a retired Colonial Governor [7]. Rae's attempt to belittle the perceptions of Eyre by the pageant as being 'cavalier' was unfortunate and indeed disingenuous, as many historical authorities thought that the the Commission's investigation into Eyre's murderous suppression of the Jamaican people at Morant Bay was a whitewash and a travesty [8].

The closing line of Rae's review expressed with some anguish '... *The case history is written up; is there no cure?...*' and is indeed a reflection of the colonized Jamaicans' perception of madness and by extension mental enslavement. *Madnificent Irations* reflected the real case study of a patient of Bellevue Hospital and its leading performer—Lockhart Hines. The production was virtually built around Hines, who played the role of the character Madman 1. A highly educated and well-trained journalist in Jamaica in the 1960s, Hines suffered repeated psychotic breakdowns for which he had been committed to Bellevue on a number of occasions. On his last admission to hospital some years previously he ended up in one of the notorious long-stay wards of the institution. The Rehabilitation

Unit that I had set up in 1974 was designed precisely to identify patients such as Lockhart, who had become sequestered in the huge custodial wards where he had become forgotten for several years and had become a shell of his former self. Designed around the concept of the therapeutic community, the Rehabilitation Unit was structured to return institutionalized patients to leading active, functional lives, performing the normal activities of daily living and encouraged to return to sustained creative vocational activity. I had selected the staff members who worked in the Unit and trained them in the art of psychiatric rehabilitation that had formed the basis of my thesis for Doctor of Medicine (Psychiatry) at the University of the West Indies. Hines had responded amazingly to this therapy and within a few months had virtually recovered from the chronic institutionalized state to which he had deteriorated. His recovery was taking place around the same time in 1977 and 1978 when the therapeutic revolution was occurring in the Bellevue Hospital and when the Garden Theatre and the cultural therapy program were being developed. The Rehabilitation Unit was located 20 yards away from the newly formed Cultural Therapy Unit and a similar distance away from the Garden Theatre that was in the process of construction. Hines put all his energy and attention into the building of the Garden Theatre and the development and writing of the *Madnificent Irations* script. His creative writing and performance skills made him the perfect choice for the role of Madman 1. He had a phenomenal memory and memorized his lines with facility and developed the creative performance with finesse and aplomb. He was a natural, and his energy was bountiful and contagious. Not only did he understand the process of madness in Jamaica, but he had lived it for much of his life.

Hines' journalistic skills were also burgeoning in parallel with his success as the male star of *Madnificent Irations*, and we were all amazed when he successfully wrote and negotiated the publication in the *Jamaica Daily News* of an account of his participation in the Bellevue Garden Theatre, the writing and development of the production of the pageant, and his own phenomenal success as the principal performer. This is reproduced below in full, courtesy of the National Library of Jamaica [9]:

> THE MORNING MIST had not yet lifted from the Blue Mountains, but one could hear the steady pounding of hammer meeting nail. The sound disturbed the birds in the Lignum Vitae overhead, and they rose as one to

find themselves a quieter haven. Not far away, a thickly muscled man, his back already wet, forced a saw through stout bamboo poles. He paused for a moment, turned to a group of men and then shouted. "Bring more come nuh man! A Thursday an opening night, you know". The men rose slowly. They seemed very tired, but they knew the task ahead. The site was bustling this Monday morning. Women were carrying bricks; men were unloading a truckfull of earth, and even children were helping with the laying of bricks for the main auditorium. As I looked around, sympathy arose in me. Something such as this – building a bamboo garden theatre would be quite a story anywhere, but I was standing in the middle of the Bellevue Hospital. How had all this come about?

Bellevue Hospital was established in 1862 at approximately the same time as Tower Street Penitentiary. This was no coincidence. The post slavery era in Jamaica was one of continuous turmoil and was marked by frequent rebellions by the newly-freed citizens. The most bloody during this time was the Morant Bay Rebellion of 1865. The rebellion brought to a head the frustrations of the newly-freed slaves, but instead of accepting the reality of equal rights for all, the colonial masters sought to create two separate societies – that of the white colonialist elite, who would still exercise illegal control over a vast majority of newly-freed slaves and their families. Up to this time, mental illness was not viewed by the white elite as a legitimate ailment which required trained personnel to undertake the care of those who suffered from various mental and emotional disorders. Prevailing idea at the time was that these disorders were incurable and the most logical reaction by the elite was to find a secure corner for the mentally ill and lock them far away. In order to reinforce the idea of incarceration Bellevue was created in the same basic design as the Tower Street Penitentiary. Of primary importance to the colonialists was security. The mentally ill, or those who were considered rebellious and therefore potentially dangerous to the establishment were locked away for life. This reveals the fundamental weakness in such a system. Many of the newly-freed, finding themselves without land or money or even the basic means for physical sustenance, vented their frustration in a variety of ways. Some found their way into the church; others sought salvation though the control of evil spirits. Still others destroyed canefields, their only means of sustenance, in an effort to register their dissatisfaction with the dictates of the elite. After the Morant Bay Rebellion, the British made cosmetic changes. They replaced Governor Eyre with another Englishman – John Peter Grant, whose methods, although in line with those of his predecessors, were not as harsh or as repressive. It should be noted that during this period no one saw fit to give the mentally disturbed protection under the law, and to this day there is no such law in Jamaica.

The conditions which led to the establishment of Bellevue moved logically to the shabby treatment of inmates and workers alike. It was not uncommon to find wards with 200 "mentally ill" individuals under one roof. Food such as yams were served unpeeled, and many wards were infested with rats, lice, and other disease-carrying pests. Very little provision was made for the basic requirements of the staff. It was a situation which cried out for attention. Dissatisfaction culminated in a strike in 1946. For three weeks the staff picketed the hospital, during which the main gates were closed to all traffic except those providing basic necessities for the patients. Dockworkers and army personnel ran the hospital, but the point was made. The strikers made two demands: (1) The removal of the Senior Medical Officer; (2) improved conditions for workers and patients. This began a workers' participation movement in the hospital. The Senior Medical Officer was a source of frustration for workers and patients alike. Up to this time, no Jamaican had held the post and the Senior Medical Officers continued the colonial tradition of seclusion and isolation for patients, and one of servitude and submissiveness for workers. Gradually conditions changed. Jamaicans could now aspire to the post of Senior Medical Officer. New categories of ancillary workers were introduced. Great importance was placed on rehabilitation as an alternative to isolation and improvement in the diet of the patients took priority. Occupational Therapy was introduced as a means of keeping the patients alert and active. The current Occupational Therapy Program began on a small scale in 1959 but has now expanded to a point where there are close to 500 paid patients out of a total population of 1800. The products of these patients vary, They make cushions, tablemats, coconut shell artefacts, handbags, knapsacks and rugs of all types. These products are sold to the public and the proceeds are used for the benefit of the patients. The post of the Senior Medical Officer is held by Dr. Fred Hickling. Dr. Hickling who has been with the Hospital for five years has been the Senior Medical Officer since last year. In that short time this reporter has seen genuine changes in the overall approach to mental illness in Bellevue. Perhaps the most striking is the development of cultural therapy. Members of this team who have specific training in the disciplines of craft, drama, speech and dance will form the core of the newest therapeutic sub-unit of the hospital – the Cultural Therapy Centre. I spoke to Dr. Hickling about the new direction that Bellevue is now taking.

Dr. Hickling, who has much experience in the fields of dance, drama and music, feels that the public has many misconceptions regarding mental illness; that the stigma of being a mental patient still hangs over the society, leading to desert their relatives who display symptoms of mental disease. The Senior Medical Officer strongly disagrees with isolation as

> a remedy, and in fact places much importance on socialization. It is this concept of integration that influenced his decision to put on a pageant of song and dance and drama in order to educate the public regarding to new approaches to mental illness. The pageant served as a means to alerting the public to their own prejudices about mental illness, raising money, involving patients, staff and community in a therapeutic exercise which was highly dependent on intergroup cooperation for its success. After deliberation with several representatives of these three general groups, rehearsal began. The script was written by Dr. Hickling and several songs and dance were contributed by the cast. Intensive rehearsals for the pageant entitled *"Madnificent Irations"* began in July. In the beginning it was felt that a temporary outdoor stage would suffice but after everyone began to "get into" their parts it appeared that nothing short of a theatre would suffice.
>
> The rest is a success story rare in our troubled land. Not only was a theatre built, but thanks to the support of the staff and the community, "Irations" is a resounding success. From the initial run of thirteen performances in two weeks the show has run for twenty-three performances in thirty days. And what of the future? As I sat with Dr Hickling in the theatre now dubbed "the Step by Step Theatre" he said with confidence, "this is just the beginning. The future looks rosy, and promising".

Lockhart Hines had conceived of and executed this beautifully constructed piece of journalism in the flush of his successful personal rehabilitation and his resounding success as the leading actor in a theatrical performance that had stunned the island of Jamaica. Who in Jamaica believed that a mad person could be rehabilitated to the point of a scintillating performance in a three-hour-long pageant in the words of his own journalism: '…a success story rare in our troubled land…'. Hines' article effectively countered and belied the concerns of Norman Rae, who had stated in his review: '*…I wish one could feel that Mad I is designed as therapy, that it might help by allowing patients to act out their frustrations publicly and so exorcise some of the demons…*'. Little did Rae know that the leading performer was a patient in the long-stay/chronic wards of Bellevue Hospital, with severe enduring mental illness, who had been incarcerated for many years in horrendous conditions in a backward asylum. That he had, through the therapeutic process of the creation of *Madnificent Irations*, been able to act out his frustrations and exorcise many of his demons, and had overcome them all with grace and composure. Hines' article addressed most of the questions posed by Rae a few weeks previously, as well as the issue of the apparently thin line between madness and sanity that Verena Reckord had remarked on in her review.

In my view it recalled the lines from Shakespeare's *Hamlet*: 'Alas poor Yorick! I knew him, Horatio: a fellow of infinite jest, of most excellent fancy'. The tragedy is that I have to say of Hines 'Alas poor Lockhart! I knew him well.' He soon was no more. Without my knowledge or consent, the senior nursing staff of the Rehabilitation Unit discharged him from hospital a few weeks after the successful run of *Madnificent Irations*, about which he had written so eloquently. After his remarkable recovery in the Rehabilitation Unit and his successful performance in the pageant, the nurse assumed he was well enough for discharge to his family home in Manchester without checking with or obtaining approval from the medical team. Such was the authority of senior nurses in Bellevue, where medical supervision was meager. Within a few weeks, Lockhart, isolated and alone, had hanged himself, a victim of the non-supportive environment he had described in his article. Few understood then or understand now the complexities of the rehabilitative care of patients with severe enduring mental illness. I doubt that the senior nurses who discharged him in 1978 were unaware of the dangers that lurked in the community for Lockhart. His social history was well known to the nursing staff. The suspicion lingered that he had been discharged out of spite—'red eye and bad mind' (jealousy related to the practice of Obeah [10])—precisely because of the adulation received following the publication of his article in the *Jamaica Daily News* and his success as the 'star performer' in *Madnificent Irations.*

The success of the cultural therapy program at Bellevue Hospital was initially documented in an article appearing in the *Journal of Hospital and Community Psychiatry* [11]. This study reported that the cohort of patients who participated in the sociodramas ($N = 38$) was compared with a control group of patients matched for age and sex ($N - 38$); mean age was 40 years, with both groups being comprised of long-stay chronic patients with a length of stay ranging from one year to 40 years, with an average of 7.6 years. The patients who participated in the sociodramas showed significantly greater decreases in medication dosage ($p < .01$) and psychosocial disability scores ($p < .001$) and significantly greater rates of improvement and discharge ($p < .001$) than patients in the control group. There was no significant difference in the diagnoses given to the two groups of patients (Fig. 7.3).

All patients in the cohort and control group were involved in hospital vocational projects, such as agricultural teams or arts and crafts manufacture, that had a high level of staff and patient participation, but only the

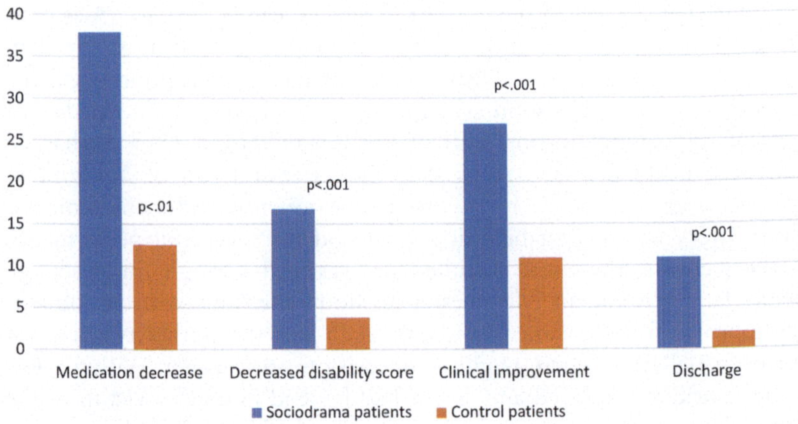

Fig. 7.3 Clinical improvements resulting from the cultural therapy program

cohort experienced the sociodrama process. The conclusion of the controlled comparison was that the significant improvement of the patients who participated in the sociodrama program could not be attributed to the intensity of staff-patient interaction that characterized the sociodrama process, but must have been a result of the process itself.

The article also described an important case study which occurred after the birth of *Madnificent Irations*, involving a young staff nurse, Arthur Miller. On one of my daily clinical meetings with the Cultural Therapy Team, I had discussed with them the world-famous experiment carried out by Stanford University professor and, psychologist David Rosenhan, that had been published in 1973, titled 'On Being Sane in Insane Places' [12]. In that experiment, eight actors had briefly feigned auditory hallucinations in the admission facilities of 12 psychiatric hospitals in five different states in the USA. All were admitted and diagnosed as having a mental illness. In spite of denying the symptoms of auditory hallucinations once they had been admitted, all had been forced to admit to being mentally ill and to take antipsychotic medication before they were granted discharge from hospital. These 'pseudo-patients' had spent an average of 19 days in hospital and were all diagnosed as being 'schizophrenic.'

This 'pseudo-patient' experiment had a profound effect on Arthur Miller. Unbeknown to me and without discussing it with anyone, he had decided to 'play-act' madness in the Bellevue Hospital one weekend when he reported for duty, by stripping off his clothes and talking loudly in a foolish and aggressive manner. He had been cruelly and forcibly restrained by some of his senior nursing colleagues and had been admitted to one of the long-stay wards of the hospital without any medical assessment or legal certification and subdued with injections of the barbiturate sodium amytal and chlorpromazine by the charge nurse on weekend duty, who acted without clinical authority and who, according to Miller, was smelling of alcohol and acting in a drunken state. After spending 2 days being forcibly incarcerated, it was reported to me as the Senior Medical Officer that Miller had been admitted to hospital. I immediately examined him and could find no evidence of mental illness. He reported to me that he had just been testing Rosenhan's 'pseudo-patient' experiment here in Bellevue. He described that he had spent most of the weekend sedated illegally, before he came to the attention of the senior nursing authorities to whom he revealed his experiment on the Monday morning following his weekend misadventure. His abnormal behavior had, by then, stopped.

At the ethnohistorical meeting following the birth of *Madnificent Irations* and the cultural therapy process, there had been an intense discussion about changing attitudes and practices in the hospital. Patients accused nurses of cruel and inhumane treatment. At one of these meetings, Miller confronted many of the older nurses, accusing them of dishonest, corrupt and hypocritical clinical and administrative practices. Their response was vehement denial. This is what had prompted Miller's 'pseudo-patient' experiment and he had anticipated the outcome. His experience of illegal admission to hospital and the undeniable illegal and cruel actions of the nurses who had admitted and subdued him silenced the senior nurses who had been seriously embarrassed by the incident. The discussion had a profound effect on the meeting participants. The incident also triggered a considerable degree of guilt in me. I realized that Miller's experiment had taken place some days after I had been teaching about Rosenhan's experiment, which appeared to have confirmed the findings of William Caudill and colleagues in the USA in the early 1950s. We had discussed this issue many times on our clinical rounds. Caudill had playacted madness and had spent 6 months in a locked mental hospital, making careful records of the injustices and dynamics of that institution [13]. Miller's boldness in replicating Rosenhan's research in Bellevue on his own was dangerous, but an act of raw courage. Some years later he completed his Ph.D. and is now a practicing drama therapist in Florida.

A recent journalistic investigative study by Susannah Cahalan [14] has severely criticized Rosenhan's 'pseudo-patient' study. She tried to track down the eight 'pseudo-patients' from the study. She interviewed two, one of whom was excluded from Rosenhan's paper because he actually liked the conditions in the mental hospital to which he had been admitted, thereby overturning Rosenhan's principal finding! I had used this article in good faith to buttress my own antipathy to custodial mental hospitals, thereby putting Miller's life at considerable risk. Fortunately for us both, the conditions at Bellevue were so poor that his courage and my observations and teachings that supported Rosenhan's research have been vindicated. However, disquiet surrounding the issue has helped create an anti-science backlash, as described by Cahalan.

Madnificent Irations was performed in front of 1500 people on the opening night at the Bellevue Garden Theatre and the players soon became famous throughout Jamaica. It was magnificent; it was 'madnificent'. The Governor-General, the Prime Minister, and high governmental officials came to the performances. All kinds of people came to see the pageant in the hospital environs. The press took it up; they just loved it. The cultural therapy program shaped a new direction for the hospital. All psychotherapeutic processes involving change generate conflict and this was no exception. The senior nurses viewed the changes taking place in the mental hospital as an abrogation of their power and therefore we had conflict relating to *ideology of custodialization*, which was the nursing staff's purview, and *work therapy*, which reflected the workers' and patients' perspective. The acting out of this conflict in the hospital generated a lot of discussion in the print media. In their newspaper articles journalists and columnists discussed the genesis of these conflicts exhaustively. As the cultural therapy process threw up different performances and different activities so did the controversy rage in the press. But the show went on, and the show did go on as the process was growing and evolving. This process was exploring our culture, our history in terms of its relationship with madness; we had fantastic talent in the mental hospital and the process was entertaining and informative. The patients became the central focus of these pageants, which were telling their stories: the madman selling the mental hospital mule, the madman advising terrified motorists on the other side of the fence.

Thousands of people from the community began attending these performances and soon the sociodrama pageants started touring Jamaica. Hilary Robertson, my partner at that time, who subsequently became my wife of 33 years, pioneered the *rural cultural engagement* of the cultural therapy process at the Staff Club of the Sugar Workers Co-operative at Bernard Lodge Sugar Estate in St. Catherine. The players piled into the hospital bus and took the performance of *Madnificent Irations* to Bernard Lodge in 1979. An audience of one thousand people each paid an entrance fee of one Jamaican dollar per person to view the performance. It was a remarkable experience! We then took the performance to the Frome Sugar Estate in the western end of Jamaica to an equally enthusiastic crowd of sugar workers as part of the worker participation program. Hilary mobilized the worker participation experimental process that had been organized at this sugar estate by the Manley government in 1977, and attracted an attentive audience of 3500 sugar workers. The constant repetitive comments of amazement from the crowd of people were: 'if they are mad people, then what about me?' The Bellevue Players, the name that the group adopted, started taking their sociodrama performances to various parts of the country. We performed the pageant in an abandoned cinema in Duckenfield, St. Thomas, a poverty-stricken area in the eastern end of the island. The technical stage team cleaned up the cinema, installed electric lighting in the building, and invited the community to an evening of madhouse entertainment.

Between 1978 and 1981, the Cultural Therapy Team at Bellevue produced four annual pageants: *Madnificent Irations*, *Visionated Penetrations*, *Madaptations*, and *Irations Explosion*. They told the story of the history of madness in a British postcolonial territory, and the genesis of mental illness in specific patients of that hospital. The pageants challenged the participants and the audiences to re-evaluate preconceived notions and stigma of 'madness' and presented visible and provocative examples of how abstract issues such as oppression, racism, madness, and conflict could be negated by the startling reality of mentally ill people performing with style and confidence in the liberating environment of the stage and the theatre. The pageants were performed to audiences within the mental hospital and all across the island, were seen by several thousands, and were reported extensively by the newspapers, television, and radio. The Cultural Therapy Team would pack up costumes and instruments, load up the bus and travel to remote areas of the island.

The team would move into a community centre or an abandoned cinema and set up performances for the rural community folk.

These pageants and the cultural therapy process had a profound effect on the mental hospital. There was a reduction in the number of conflicts among patients, staff, and administrators, an increased focus on productivity, and improved communication and changes in therapeutic attitudes and practices. There was a threefold decrease in the use of medication and significant decrease in psychosocial disability scores for patients who participated in the process compared with non-participant controls, and a very significant increase in a positive clinical outcome of the participants compared with the controls [11]. By 1979, hundreds of patients daily were being exposed to the programs at the Cultural Therapy Centre.

By that time, the Edna Manley Cultural Training Centre (now the Edna Manley College of the Visual and the Performing Arts (EMCVPA)) had begun to recognize the importance of these programs and was beginning to train its own students in the use of culture as therapy to be used not only in the mental health field but in prisons and other institutional settings. Journalist Curtis Myrie, in a report published in the *Jamaica Daily News* in April 1979, described the placement of five second-year students (Michael Smith, Mataoumba Nyahuma, Paul Pinto, Juliet Smith and Delores Williams) attending the School of Drama at Bellevue in an internship training program. Organized by EMCVPA faculty Dennis Scott and Hortencer Lindsay, it was designed to expose the students to the cultural therapy program at Bellevue. A number of these interns went on to play pivotal roles in establishing successful cultural therapy programs in Jamaican prisons such as the Gun Court. Michael Smith played a major role in the development of the Gun Court cultural therapy movement, which won a number of awards.

Many British psychiatrists privately suggest that psychotherapy is not appropriate for minority groups because of their supposed lack of 'verbal facility' or the ability to understand and 'work through' their problems in a way that accords with the psychological model [15]. Littlewood makes it clear that many British psychiatrists and psychotherapists have rejected this position as racist, expressing his opposition to the view [16]. The Rastafarian neologism *overstand* poses a dialectical antithetical construct, carrying the phonological implication of the root word 'understand' into a new context, representing the antipodal reality to Littlewood's limited insight. The realities of *Madnificent Irations* and this cultural therapy experience force the *overstanding* of the ego-centric global psychological issues of these Western psychiatric perceptions that have been based on racism born out of centuries of colonial misadventure. This semiotic process is central to the application of cultural therapy.

There is no doubt that Bellevue was locked in the throes of a huge cultural therapy experiment which equated to the practice of psychotherapy, in the broadest sense. Specific psychotherapeutic activities had been instituted for all members of the total institution. A clear progression had emerged. Contradictions had been engaged and a fierce struggle of opposing forces or vectors had surfaced. The resultant transformation not only produced visible changes and products, but also unleashed violent opposition and cataclysmic resistance. Not all the inhabitants of the total institution were happy, or pleased with the direction of the change. Most of those dissatisfied with the process were the professional nurses, nursing administrators, and their allies. They perceived the changes as being unprofessional, non-medical, and most importantly, that the changes had wrenched the supreme authority of the institution from their hands into the hands of the underclass.

In an article published in *Interventions* in 2004, I identified that the use of culture as an instrument for education, consciousness-raising, and demystification, as well as entertainment, is a tool which the peoples of the world have been using in the struggle for freedom, land, and better working conditions for centuries and has been rediscovered and titled people's (or popular) theatre in recent years [17]. The development of an active popular theatre movement in Jamaica intensified in the 1970s, building on the foundation established by Marcus Garvey at Edelweiss Park in Kingston in the early 1910s. Garvey insisted that Black Jamaicans must provide an arena for their creative expression in drama, music, and poetry. Edelweiss Park provided that opportunity, allowing Jamaican artists and performers to express their creativity (and get paid for doing so) on a regular basis. In the context of colonial Jamaica at the time, this was revolutionary and laid the foundation for the development of contemporary theatre.

Bibliography

1. Hickling FW (1985) Poem "Westminster System" (Unpublished).
2. Reckord V (1978) Madnificent Irations—Well Worth Watching. *Jamaica Daily News*, September 13, 1978. The *Jamaica Daily News* was published in Kingston 1973–1983. After its closure it was publicly archived at The National Library of Jamaica. https://www.instituteofjamaica.org.jm/.

3. *The Daily Gleaner* of Tuesday September 5, 1978.
4. Nana (1978) “Mi mad? Yu mussi mad!”, *Jamaica Daily News*, September 24.
5. Milner H (1982) *The Daily Gleaner*, Thursday, September 9.
6. Rae N (1978) column “A Line from the Tower of Babble: Madnificent Irations at the Bellevue Garden Theatre”, *Gleaner*, September 10.
7. McLintock AH (Ed.) (2009) ‘EYRE, Edward John’, from *An Encyclopaedia of New Zealand*, originally published in 1966. Te Ara—The Encyclopaedia of New Zealand. Consulted 22 April 2009. http://www.TeAra.govt.nz/en/1966/eyre-edward-john.
8. Handford P (2008) Edward John Eyre and the Conflict of Laws. *Melbourne University Law Review, 32*(3), 822–860.
9. Hines L (1978) The Future Looks Rosy. *Jamaica Daily News*, October 20.
10. Hickling FW, James C (2008) ‘Traditional Mental Health Practices in Jamaica: On the Phenomenology of Red Eye, Bad Mind and Obeah’. In FW Hickling, BM Mathies, KA Morgan, RC Gibson (Eds.), *Perspectives in Caribbean Psychology*. Kingston: CARIMENSA Press, University of the West Indies Mona.
11. Hickling FW (1989) Sociodrama in the Rehabilitation of Chronic Mentally Ill Patients. *Hospital and Community Psychiatry, 40*, 402–406.
12. Rosenhan D (1973) On Being Sane in Insane Places. *Science, 179* (4070), 250–258.
13. Caudill W, Redlich FC, Gilmore HR, Brody E et al. (1952) Social Structure and Interaction Processes on a Psychiatric Ward. *American Journal of Orthopsychiatry, 22*, 314–334.
14. Cahalan S (2019) *The Great Pretender: The Undercover Mission That Changed Our Understanding of Madness*. New York, Boston: Grand Central Publishing.
15. Kareem J, Littlewood R (Eds.) (1992) *Intercultural Therapy: Themes, Interpretations and Practice*. Oxford. Blackwell.
16. Littlewood R (1992) Towards an Intercultural Therapy. In J Kareem, R Littlewood (Eds.), *Intercultural Therapy: Themes, Interpretations and Practice*. Oxford. Blackwell.
17. Hickling FW (2004) Popular Theatre as Psychotherapy. *Interventions: International Journal of Post-Colonial Studies, 6*(1), 45–56.

CHAPTER 8

Political Sequelae: Destruction of the Garden Theatre

For is him create Westminster
That keeps us still enslaved
To the coattail of him dunza
An to an image which he made. [1]

The struggle for political power, as a conscious reflection of decolonization and class struggle, brought Jamaica to the brink of civil war by the end of 1980. The hidden agenda that surfaced in post-emancipation colonial Jamaica in 1938 in the labor riots of that time [2] was buried soon again with the emergence of the Jamaica Labour Party (JLP) in 1943 as a contender for power against the People's National Party (PNP), which was the original political formation of the 1938 Jamaican National Liberation Movement. No doubt Sir Arthur Richards, the British Colonial Governor at that time, secretly congratulated himself on the success of his 'divide and rule' strategy when a founder member of the PNP, and a leader of the National Liberation Movement, Alexander Bustamante, was released from four years of political detention in 1942 [3]. Bustamante had been detained in 1939 by Richards on the order of the Colonial Office in London, after making extremely radical and revolutionary speeches to striking cane workers [4]. He stormed out of the PNP, which he had helped to form, and created the objective conditions for the resurgence of the hidden agenda. By setting up the JLP in 1943, Bustamante effectively divided the National Liberation Movement and turned brother against brother. This was in accordance with one

F. W. Hickling, *Decolonization of Psychiatry in Jamaica*,
https://doi.org/10.1007/978-3-030-48489-7_8

of the hallmarks of British colonialism—the process of divide and rule. Objectively the same struggle split the country again by 1980. Class conflict, simmering uneasily as the hidden decolonial agenda was intensified by the democratic socialist platform of the PNP of the 1970s, was documented by Michael Manley as the struggle to move the Jamaican people out of the clutches of the world capitalist system, in search of a new economic order [5]. The class struggle that raged was reflected in the power struggle between individuals, men and women, families, and institutions. The most obvious example of this was the struggle for political power, adhering to the Westminster model bequeathed by the British colonizers as they withdrew, following confrontation by the people in 1938.

The practice of psychiatry in Jamaica in the decade of the 1970s was challenging and revealing. The political events of the time forced even the most cautious and most conservative to look closely at the behavior of people in and out of the consulting room in the context of the concurrent social events. The violence and aggression posed a particular dilemma, requiring the application of solutions at all therapeutic levels and critical examination of prevailing attitudes and trends within institutions. Psychiatrists were being forced to deal with and find solutions to multiple and repeated incidences of psychosociological problems such as violence, crime, poverty, and unemployment, which formed the backdrop to the multifaceted, neoliberal cultural expression of religious and educational norms appearing in the wider society at that time. Psychosis, drug abuse, psychopathic behavior, and institutionalized repression were all symptomatic of the psychopathology of the times and psychiatrists were forced to develop and test solutions to help combat them. No doubt the experience at Bellevue Hospital involving employment of even the most severely enduring mentally ill person was a significant challenge. The establishment of therapeutic communities heralding new approaches of collective democracy with a flattening of the authority pyramid inherited from the slave plantation and the introduction of the concept of productivity circles at all levels of work organization, cut across the established and rigidly held hierarchical organization of a colonial custodial system. The provision of cultural therapy and sociodrama as instruments for large-scale institutional psychotherapy, community engagement in the form of out-patient clinics, social work intervention, family therapy, counseling services, and psychotherapy, represented tangible manifestations of that blueprint which psychiatrists were being forced to write. Clearly, Michael Manley thought that there was a need for this approach, as he tried to implement a political solution through the vehicle of democratic socialism and the PNP. In *Jamaica: Struggle in the Periphery* published in 1983, Manley describes the socio-political therapeutic measures introduced by his administration in the attempt to achieve resolution to the contradictions of this complex Jamaican society [5]. Asserting that although the program was not a radical one, he agreed that these measures brought Jamaica to the verge of a civil war.

Political insight was to play an extremely important role in the process of political decolonization of the mental hospital and of the minds of the people of Jamaica at that critical juncture in its history. In the general election of 1976 the PNP, employing the rhetoric of democratic socialism, received an overwhelming plebiscite to carry out a program of political transformation. Manley's government became increasingly close to the Cuban government of Fidel Castro. One of the showcases of the Castro regime was the organizational and vocational productivity on display at the Havana Psychiatric Hospital.

In my visits to Cuba in 1974 and 1977, I had been overwhelmed by the incredible display of activities at the hospital, which ranged from the upkeep of the largest rose garden in Cuba to organized sports, including baseball and basketball. There was also a wide range of entertainment and cultural activity. For a psychiatrist from the dilapidated dungeon which was Bellevue Hospital at that time, it was a revelation. I could only gaze in astonishment. Manley and his colleagues had visions of Bellevue being transformed in a similar manner and felt that they now had the opportunity to make that happen. So it was not surprising, when I submitted my official request to recruit additional medical personnel, that Michael should turn to his friend Fidel. The response was almost immediate. The Cuban government started sending psychiatrists to Jamaica to help with the psychiatric transformatory work that had started in the mid-1960s. Between 1977 and 1980, I benefited from the assistance of sixteen Cuban psychiatrists who worked at Bellevue, and in the Community Psychiatric Service in the parish of Westmoreland. The Cubans played an extremely important role in helping to establish the work therapy program at Bellevue and made an effective contribution to the process of psychohistoriographic cultural therapy and community engagement that had been instituted in the early 1970s.

After the change of government following the devastating electoral defeat of the PNP in 1980, many of the gains which had been made by the mental health movement in the previous decade, including the process of decentralization and the transformation of Bellevue, were drastically reversed. There was an almost complete return to the anti-therapeutic custodial mode of care in the institution. In 1984, the therapeutic community activities were stopped. The Bellevue Garden Theatre, including the exquisite handiwork of several hundred severely mentally ill patients, was demolished (Fig. 8.1). The Cultural Therapy Centre was disbanded and the team members who had been specially trained for this purpose at the Edna Manley College for the Visual and Performance Arts were returned to routine custodial ward activities in the 24 long-stay wards of the hospital.

The destruction of the Garden Theatre and the eradication of the cultural therapy process were carried out in a particularly vicious and vindictive manner, which defied logic and rational explanation. A bulldozer was employed to push down the bamboo walls, remove the seating and flatten the site. The Jamaica Popular Theatre Alliance (JAPTA)

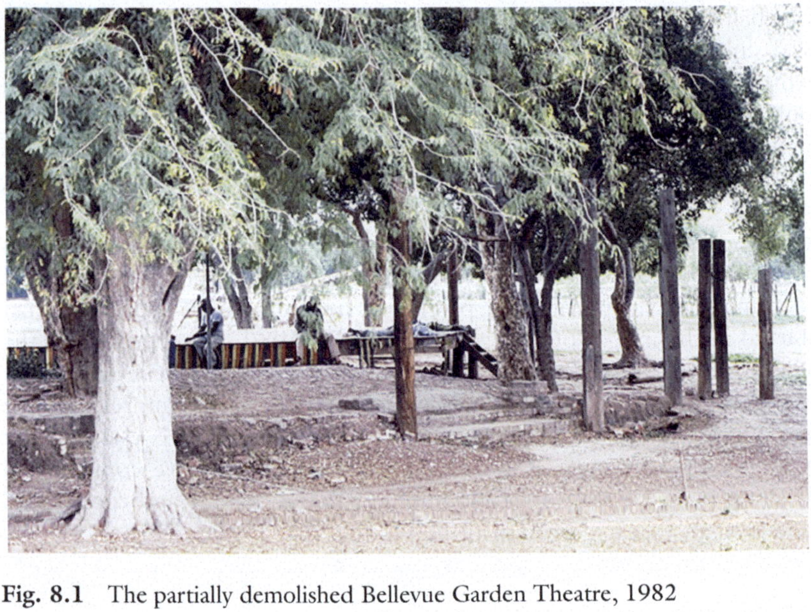

Fig. 8.1 The partially demolished Bellevue Garden Theatre, 1982

protested that the theatre had been demolished. The hospital management explained that the bamboo had deteriorated over the years; that the area was being misused at night for criminal and gambling activities and that the theatre was being abused by bad elements. Veteran theatre critic Archie Lindo in his weekly column in *The Star* wrote:

> I was rather upset to read in the press about the 'tearing down' of the Bellevue Bamboo Theatre. Mind you there are always two sides to every story. I do know that Dr. Hickling had a good idea when he set up and built that theatre. The therapy value on patients was immense and he did stage quite a few successes with patients and staff acting together. I know that bamboo does not last long as building material. Sometimes it rots quite easily and has to be replaced. But it would be quite a pity if the Bellevue Theatre was torn down and 'put away' completely. I do not know all the facts. But what I do feel is that some agreement, and a pleasant one at that can be reached if there was a get-together of the big-people in this thing, a talk-out and an eventual agreement on the lines to be taken on something like this. Replace the old bamboo with well-prepared well-treated bamboo. Invite Dr. Hickling to the conference on the subject and work out something. When the new Theatre is built, it would be a good, and friendly, gesture to invite him to attend the opening ceremony, and actually be the one to declare the new Theatre open. Dr. Hickling not only had the idea for the Theatre but he had it built and put on several plays (mainly for therapy treatment) but which were also enjoyed by members of the public as well as by the members of the cast (including Staff and patients). He himself wrote the scripts and there was even a nice little musical band accompanying the cast. As I have already mentioned the venture was a success from many points of view and it would be a pity to 'lose' it all. I would be very glad to see some agreement reached. If we set our minds to it a well-arranged meeting could settle the whole thing and it could be righted-out once more from there. How about it all concerned? The venture is a worthwhile one and it would be a pity to lose it entirely. [6]

Lindo's commentary was a 'give away' of the intense political conflict that was raging behind the scenes between the conservative JLP of which Seaga was the leader and Prime Minister, and the democratic socialist PNP, for whom the Bellevue Garden Theatre was regarded as something of a victorious 'socialist icon' of the previous government. The commentary positioned Archie Lindo as a mediator, an elder statesman of the theatre, trying to 'calm the troubled waters' and if possible emerge with a conciliatory settlement. Twice in the commentary Lindo wrote of the concept of 'the loss' of the theatre and the process that emerged, and the idea that with a 'well-arranged' 'get-together' of the 'big-people' a 'talk-out and an eventual agreement' could be reached. Lindo's attempt at political reconciliation was, however, a sad joke, given that memories of the 800 people who had been killed in the near civil war between the two political parties that had accompanied the political election of 1980 were still fresh. In an article in the *New York Times* in 1988, Mark Kurlansky described Edward Seaga as a 'pragmatist criticized even within in his party for cold-bloodedness…' [7]. Kurlansky described the rivalry between the JLP and PNP as 'clanlike,' not ideological, demanding 'ironclad loyalty which they pay off with patronage,' which has been the root of the tribal violence in Jamaica.

The hospital administration's rationale for the demolition of the theatre—the deterioration of the bamboo over the years, as described by Lindo—was disingenuous at least and dishonest at best, as the walls and seating were always replaced when they showed signs of deterioration, as part of the vocational strategy of the hospital therapeutic rehabilitation program. The reality was that the week that I departed the institution, the cultural therapy activities in the center were stopped, and, as mentioned above, the Cultural Therapy Team members were reassigned to the numerous hospital long-stay wards. Many of them subsequently resigned and migrated to the USA. Team members like 'Big J' Johnson and Ruddy Rennocks quickly found employment in New York. When last I heard from him, former staff nurse Arthur Miller had completed his Ph.D. and was pursuing a successful drama therapy career in Florida. Others, like Valrette Kirkland, Neila Johnson, Joe Williams, and Gilbert Binns, resumed custodial nursing functions at Bellevue.

As Senior Medical Officer (SMO) and a civil servant I could not be fired from Bellevue, but I was immediately transferred to a parochial rural hospital in the parish of Trelawny, deep in Cockpit country, called Ulster Spring Hospital. This was tantamount to being banished to Siberia in the Soviet Union! I resigned forthwith and established a private psychiatric practice in Kingston. I remembered the fate of my grand-uncle, Dr. Hopetoun Edward Bond, who had resigned as Acting SMO at the asylum, having been demoted at the end of World War I. I set up my practice in Connolley House, a building that had been purchased by my grandfather Frederick Pape Bond, after he had been demoted as Acting Attorney General in the Jamaica Crown Colony, also at the end of World War I. One of the stalwarts of the Cultural Therapy Team, Sonia Swaby, resigned her post as psychiatric nursing aide to become my receptionist, a post that she held for several years before migrating to the USA.

Why destroy a creative productive process that clearly empowers the liberation of mentally helpless people and provides the basis for their rise out of the poverty that enslaved them? Even the most partisan political zealot recognized the strengths of the process. The action only makes sense within the dialectical response to the 'European psychosis' in the Jamaican context. The liberating potential of this profound cultural therapy process so fundamentally challenged and threatened the survival of the conceptual European hegemony in practice that it had to be ruthlessly destroyed. The paradox is that the new Prime Minister, Edward Seaga, had instituted all of these public policy changes in what seemed to be an irrational personal vendetta and illogical response toward the progress which had been made in the institution.

The ostensible justification for the destruction of the Bellevue Garden Theatre and the cultural therapy movement seemed very, very clear to me, although nobody ever came out and said it; few people came out and said anything. Archie Lindo in his commentary came the closest to describing the profound conflicts that underpinned the destruction of the theatre. The SMO who replaced me at Bellevue Hospital following my resignation presided over the destruction of the Garden Theatre, as well as the dismantling of the Cultural Therapy Team and the Therapeutic Community Rehabilitation program. My resignation was prompted by the appointment of a Chief Nursing Officer (CNO) by the Ministry of Health, whom I had strongly recommended against hiring. The CNO was one of the nurses in Bellevue Hospital who had openly and vigorously opposed the establishment and functioning of the Cultural Therapy Centre and the Therapeutic Community Rehabilitation program at the hospital. Some of the senior nurses viewed the therapeutic community changes taking place in the mental hospital as an abrogation of their power.

The resulting conflict, as mentioned in the previous chapter, related to the *ideology of custodialization*, which was the nursing staff's purview, and *work therapy*, which was the workers' and patients' perspective. There was an active faction at the hospital advocating the return of the hospital to a conservative custodial function that was favored by the prevailing neoliberal JLP government. I resigned from my post in acknowledgment that our opposing clinical principles would have resulted in irrevocable administrative conflict that would have been impossible to contain.

I later confronted my successor about his role in what subsequently happened. We were at a private party hosted by an American psychiatrist who was a member of the Black Psychiatrists of America, during an American Psychiatric Association meeting in Los Angeles in 1984. He said that the Ministry of Health people thought that patients were smoking ganja at the Garden Theatre and that was why the program had been stopped. Furthermore, the Garden Theatre was slated to be rebuilt at another site within the grounds of the Bellevue Hospital. I retorted that ganja smoking was endemic in Bellevue and that patients and staff had been smoking ganja at the hospital since the beginning of its existence. I believe my successor was articulating the official line, but what actually happened in a public policy sense was that it allowed the JLP government to dismantle the process of what they saw as a Cuban socialist model of transformation of the hospital. This was nonsense, of course, as the transformation of the 1970s was planned and engineered by Jamaican people, long before the flirtation with Cuban politics by Michael Manley and the PNP. We received some clinical assistance from a small team of psychiatrists from Cuba for a period of four years. Seaga was paranoid about this. His actions indicated that anything related to the democratic socialist policies of the PNP, particularly any collaboration with Cuba, had to be expunged from the map of Jamaican society, regardless of whether it was successful, whether it had been proved to work and whether the country had benefited from the process. This political paranoia was expressed all over the country and not only were programs that had even a hint of the previous government's political flirtations expunged from the political map, but in the context of Bellevue, Seaga forced the reintroduction of the former colonial model of custodialization for dealing with madness; by locking patients up, scraping them up off the streets. That's why to this day the JLP is powerfully ambivalent about the community mental health movement and about attempts to deinstitutionalize Bellevue. There are deep-seated psychological prejudices that are held about the way in which mad people should be dealt with and treated. No doubt there were also personal animosities that were felt toward me owing to my enthusiastic, albeit not uncritical, support of the PNP government's agenda and opposition to the policies of the JLP.

A similar atmosphere of paranoia surrounded the community engagement and health education sphere of the mental health revolution. In 1975, when the cultural therapy decolonization program was set up at Bellevue, I participated in a community radio program, titled 'At Home' (later 'Taking Care of Business'), that went out every Thursday morning on the government-owned Jamaica Broadcasting Corporation (JBC). I was the 'Radio Psychiatrist in the morning' [8]. The program was the idea of an extremely talented broadcaster, Beverley Cole. The radio psychiatrist received telephone calls from people all over the island and answered questions raised in letters by writers who did not have access to a telephone. Callers were advised as to the possible causes of their problems, and there were discussions of the social, psychological, and psychiatric issues that had been raised. Callers were also referred to agencies or therapists where they could obtain help. There were, in addition, diagnostic evaluations, the dispensing of therapeutic advice and referrals. Figure 8.2 depicts the psychotherapeutic process. The radio psychiatrist assesses the mental status of callers while he converses with them. Psychosomatic symptoms, headaches, bodily aches and pains, and gynecological problems are described, leading in turn to discussions on psychological dependency, unconscious conflicts, and socio-economic problems, which are analyzed in terms of race, sex, power, religion and social class.

The program ran for nearly ten years, once per week initially, but became so popular that another weekly one hour slot was added some years later, featuring a second psychiatrist. I was happy for the introduction of another psychiatrist on the program as it afforded the listening public alternative psychiatric interpretations and opinions, and broadened the scope of the program and its efficacy. There was always a non-medical presenter on the program who would introduce the callers and act as a bridge or a buffer between them and the radio psychiatrist. Beverley Cole was replaced in due course by Elaine Wint, who went on to host the program for several years. At the same time, the title of the program was changed to 'Taking Care of Business'. Another popular Jamaican radio personality, Fay Ellington, also hosted the program during this period. This program brought psychiatry to the people and soon became extremely popular. It was aired at prime time in the morning when most people were traveling to work or just beginning their day. The callers often requested information on extremely delicate topics, and the psychiatrist's responses were frank and open, but sensitive.

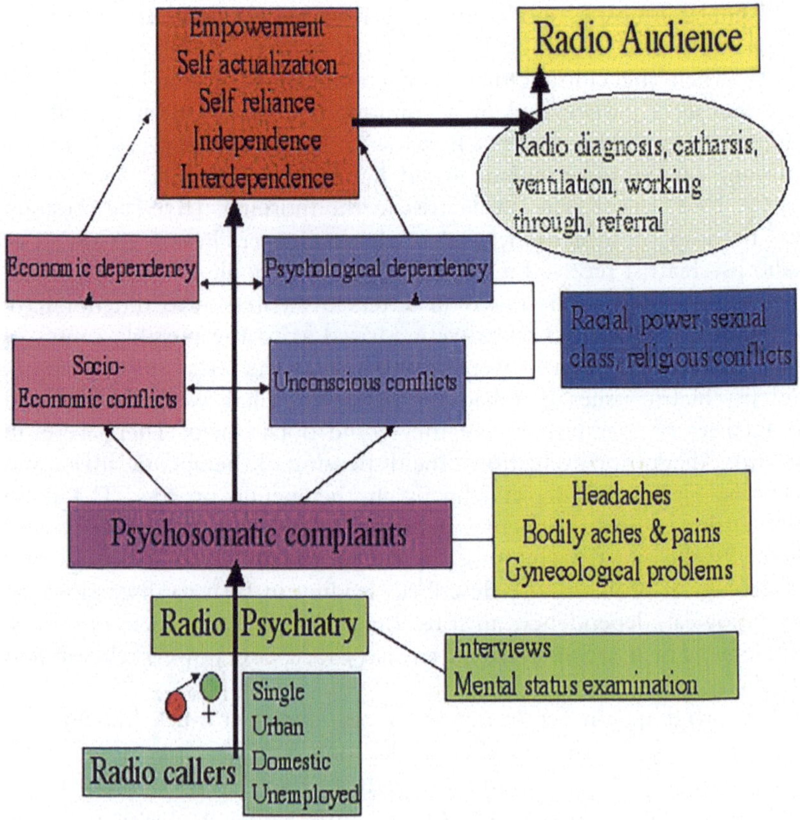

Fig. 8.2 Radio psychotherapy

The 150 programs that aired between March 1980 and February 1984 were recorded and studied. In total, 367 calls and 171 letters were received during that period, 81% of them from women. The psychiatrist spent an average of 12 minutes with each caller, and more than 50% of calls were at least 10 minutes in duration. The majority of callers were single, and included domestic helpers, unemployed persons, and students. A total of 77% of the group called about matters concerning their own mental health [8]. The radio psychiatry program answered a large number of telephone calls and letters and had a tremendous listenership as was confirmed by the listenership surveys carried out at the time. The program was extraordinarily successful, positively influencing people who called in with mild to severe clinical problems. Callers and listeners expressed positively while on air that the program had helped them and had increased their understanding of mental illness. Media surveys carried out in 1977, 1979 and 1981 indicated that it had one of the highest listenerships of all programs of a similar length and regularly attracted audiences of 120,000, in an island with a population of 2 million [9–11]. This represented a total of 58% of the national listenership, the highest sustained percentage for any 45-minute JBC program. In addition, the listenership extended as far as Florida. A survey of 100 informants conducted by the University of the West Indies in 1985 suggested that the program had a long-lasting positive effect on the community and helped a high percentage of people mentioned in the case studies in dealing with their mental health problems [12].

In an article in *Time* Magazine, [13] the establishment of the first radio psychiatry program in the USA in California in 1976 was reported, while the growing popularity of these programs in the USA and elsewhere was noted [14]. The establishment of a similar program on NBC Radio in New York in 1982 was also described [15]. It is worth noting in this context that it was Jamaica, a developing country, which pioneered the format in 1975. While it was technically similar to the programs in the USA, both the population it reached and the mental health concerns it addressed were significantly different, even though the diagnostic categories were similar. The Jamaican callers were from a lower socioeconomic class, had consistently more socioeconomic concerns and interpersonal conflicts. The psychiatric interventions in Jamaica required more than twice the average length of call as the New York program and were able to resolve significantly more of the problems and concerns on air. It was my experience on the Jamaican program that the technical producers from the radio network tried to reduce the length of time spent with each caller in the interests of commercial viability and the need to increase the number of advertisements aired. The longest time spent with any one caller on the Jamaican program was 42 minutes. It is suggested that in the commercial climate of many of the North American-based radio psychiatry programs at the time that similar resolution of mental health problems in a psychodynamic manner on air was infrequently attempted due to commercial time constraints.

On many occasions on the Jamaican program extremely distressed and seemingly suicidal patients were dealt with on air, often with a relief of the distress by the end of the call, and resolution of the problem by self-determination mutually agreed to by caller and therapist. Feedback from listeners indicated that many were satisfied by the resolution of the problem on air. People commenting on the program often suggested that the process of working through problems with callers helped listeners to address and resolve the problems they were experiencing themselves. On many occasions, listeners called into the program to express these experiences on the air. Occasionally, mental health workers in different areas all over the island called the program to report that patients who had been referred to them by the program had actually attended and had received the appropriate care and had made a satisfactory recovery.

On January 26, 1984, I was fired by the JBC in the middle of a broadcast. The letter of dismissal was placed in front of me. I opened it, read its contents to the listening audience, and bid them farewell. This was probably at the instigation of the political figures who had engineered my departure from Bellevue and given the order to bulldoze the Garden Theatre. The story made front-page headlines of *The Star* the following Tuesday:

> Popular Kingston Psychiatrist Dr. Fred Hickling was fired by the JBC Thursday, while he was on the air talking with callers. "I was most surprised and taken aback on Thursday January 26, when I, as it were, was fired on the air while moderating the popular JBC Radio programme, 'Taking Care of Business'", the popular psychiatrist told the *Star*. "I was quite surprised", he said "because the letter stating the [termination] of my service 'as of this moment' gave no reason as to whether I had done anything wrong or said anything to hurt or upset anyone". Dr. Hickling had been filling the psychiatric slot on this JBC programme since October 1975. The programme had started as 'At Home', with Beverley Cole, and in 1977–78 it became 'Taking Care of Business' with Elaine Wint as the moderator from 8.45 to 9.30 each weekday. Dr. Hickling was the psychiatrist in that slot every Thursday morning.... Speaking with the *Star* about the abrupt termination of his service on the programme, Dr. Hickling said that at about 9.20 Thursday morning while he was speaking with a caller a letter addressed to him was placed before him "terminating my service at that moment. I was quite taken by surprise. After the program ended, I just left. When you are fired you are just fired". Asked by the *Star* about the

> firing of Dr. Hickling on the air, Mr. Desmond Elliott, supervisor of the radio division of the JBC said that the corporation was making changes for improvement both at the parent and the regional stations. The letter to Dr. Hickling had stated that his (Dr. Hickling's) service was being terminated for the time being. … Dr. Hickling feels that he was taken off TCB [Taking Care of Business] unceremoniously. Several people have expressed disgust at the manner in which he was told of the termination for his service on the programme, which they say is important to members of the public. Dr. Hickling had been Senior Medical Officer of the Bellevue Hospital. [16]

I have always assumed that the order to fire was influenced by Seaga, the de facto head of the government-owned broadcasting company. There is no doubt that the mental health service in Jamaica had undergone a radical transformation in the previous two decades, and that the radio psychiatry program and the cultural therapy program at Bellevue Hospital had significantly facilitated this transformation. The population of the only state mental hospital had been reduced by nearly two-thirds over a ten-year period; the pattern of care of the acutely ill had been radically changed. The majority of mentally ill persons in Jamaica were now being treated at home, at community clinics, and at public and private general hospitals around the island. The quality of psychiatric care rose significantly in the country, and the stigma toward mental illness fell dramatically [17, 18].

However, these hostile political reactions had come too late: the genie was already out of the bottle. The Jamaican people were beginning to 'overstand' the psychic and political significance of the decolonization struggle and were beginning to 'own their own madness' [19]. Mental illness is no longer feared in the way that it was, is discussed openly on radio talk shows, and patients are comfortable to receive treatment for a variety of psychiatric conditions in community treatment facilities all over the island. Certainly, the level of violence and aggression in the acutely mentally ill has fallen dramatically in recent years. No longer are patients arrested by the police and brought tied hand and foot to treatment centers; straitjackets and canvas camisoles are things of the past. Decolonizing mental health strategies has challenged the lie, promulgated for 60 years, about the value of the two-party system foisted upon Jamaica by the colonial government and maintained by a marriage between the plantocracy and certain sections of the working-class movement. Politicians at home and abroad have exploited this situation to split the political movement for decolonization and freedom of the Jamaican people, which has, in turn, led to the virulent societal violence that has afflicted this country in recent decades. This political formation has also led to the problems of underdevelopment: the political and economic impoverishment that we are living through. Most importantly people in the country were beginning to have insight about the psychic power struggle that was at the heart of their lives and was at the core of their historical origins in the New World. They had also begun to get a glimpse of the terrible fear which the European-American psychosis had created surrounding the quest for freedom of people of color and were developing strategies and tools to negate it. The post-independence decolonizing mental health programs that had been engineered in Jamaica were bringing insight to the people about the socio-political causes of their mental illnesses, accompanied by strategies to improve their mental health.

The psychiatrists in Jamaica remain divided on partisan political issues, like the rest of society, although they have managed to work together on the practical implementation of the collective clinical principles of management. It is in the areas of religious and political ideology that the differences are greatest and have led to uncomfortable contradictions and polarities. Postcolonial Jamaican society has demanded that the psychiatrists provide the strategies for the understanding of people's behavior and help to write the prescription for individual and social change. Perhaps the psychiatrists' main task in postcolonial Jamaica and the Caribbean is to broaden understanding of power struggles and the challenge of managing authority. The defiance and conflict resulting from the imposition of governmental authority and the lack of personal autonomy are endemic in Jamaican society [20]. This must certainly be the main challenge for the future. The cultural therapy movement pioneered at the Bellevue Hospital is a postcolonial strategy designed, at its core, to challenge the colonial delusions which have engineered the oppression and self-destructive behavior of Caribbean people. Journalist Glen Bowen, writing in 1982 about the powerful effect of the cultural therapeutic decolonizing process instituted at Bellevue, believed that the 'action of the Bellevue staff in the 1970s, led by Senior Medical Officer Freddie Hickling, to create a revolution at the hospital left very little to be desired' [21]. He suggested that the hospital's work therapy and cultural therapy programs that were at the heart of the rehabilitation thrust were working wonders.

Bibliography

1. Hickling FW (1985) Poem "Westminster System" (Unpublished).
2. Hart R (2006) *The End of Empire: Transition to Independence in Jamaica and Other Caribbean Region Colonies*. Kingston: Arawak Press.
3. Richards A (1940) Letter to Secretary of State for the Colonies from Governor of Jamaica. Extract: C.O.137/840/68551229/8788 d/d 13/9/40.
4. Hickling FW, Gibson RC (2005) Philosophy and Epistemology of Caribbean Psychiatry. In FW Hickling, E Sorel (Eds.), *Images of Psychiatry: The Caribbean*. Department of Community Health and Psychiatry. Mona: University of the West Indies.
5. Manley M (1983) *Jamaica: Struggle in the Periphery*. London: Writers and Readers.
6. Lindo A (1984) Theatre Chatter—Bellevue Theatre. *The Star*, March 9.
7. Kurlansky M (1988) Showdown in Jamaica. *The New York Times Magazine*, November 27, p. 48.
8. Hickling FW (1992) Radio Psychiatry and Community Mental Health. *Hospital and Community Psychiatry, 43*, 739–741.
9. Jamaica Media Survey (1977) Kingston: Market Research Services.
10. Jamaica Media Survey (1979) Kingston: Market Research Services.
11. Jamaica Media Survey (1981) Kingston: Market Research Services.
12. Johansen M (1985) *A Questionnaire Survey of a Radio Psychiatry Program in Jamaica*, BA thesis (Mass Communications), University of the West Indies, Mona, Jamaica.
13. Cave R (1980) Dial Dr Tony for Therapy. *Time* Magazine, May 26.
14. Rice B (1981) Call-In Therapy: Reach Out and Shrink Someone. *Psychology Today*, December, pp. 39–41.
15. Ruben HL (1986) Reflections of a Radio Psychiatrist. *Hospital and Community Psychiatry, 37*, 934–936.
16. Proute JC (1984) Fired on the Air. *The Star*, Kingston, Jamaica, January 31.
17. Gibson RC, Abel WD, White S, Hickling FW (2008). Internalizing Stigma Associated with Mental Illness: Findings from a General Population Survey in Jamaica. *Pan American Journal of Public Health, 23*(1), 26–32.
18. Hickling FW, Robertson-Hickling HA, Paisley V (2011). Deinstitutionalization and Attitudes Toward Mental Illness: A Qualitative Study. *Revista Panamericana de Salud Publica/Pan American Journal of Public Health, 29*(3), 169–176.
19. Hickling FW (2020) Owning Our Madness: Contributions of Jamaican Psychiatry to Decolonizing Global Mental Health. *Transcultural Psychiatry, 57*(1), 19–31.
20. Hickling FW, Hutchinson G (2012) Madness as Social Defiance in African Caribbean Youth: Evidence from the Dancehall. *Wadabagei: A Journal of the Caribbean and Its Diasporas, 13*(3), 3–25.
21. Bowen G (1982) *The Jamaica Daily News*, December 24.

CHAPTER 9

Poetic Poiesis and Cultural Therapy

Mek we bruck out of de shackles
That still keeps our minds enslaved
Like Procrustes an fe him long bed
Who stretched each man from toe to head. [1]

The process of psychological decolonization requires a seminal 'overstanding' (Rastafarian phonological inversion of 'understanding') of the *slave mind* and the *backra massa* (slavemaster) mind and the complex integrative relationship between them. What happens to the collective mind of a people forcibly ripped from their homes and families, transported at gunpoint like cattle, shipped across thousands of miles of tempestuous oceans and enslaved on cruel plantations in a strange land? What happens to the psyche of the descendants of this African people enslaved in the New World when their language and their music, their poetry and their songs are cold-bloodedly eradicated, ruthlessly and demoniacally erased by marauding armies of slavers? What machinations occur in the minds of a race of people besotted by a delusional belief in the supremacy of their white skin? What leads them to determine that all other races with skin of varying hues can be deemed to be subhuman and their persons and possessions confiscated in fits of genocidal rage and destruction, in the belief that 'all that I see is mine, and all belongs to me; your land, your property, your husbands and your wives'? What happens to the lives and culture of the descendants of these people of color who are forced to labor without pay, for inhuman hours at the end

F. W. Hickling, *Decolonization of Psychiatry in Jamaica*,
https://doi.org/10.1007/978-3-030-48489-7_9

of a whip, and who are sadistically tortured by monstrous unrelenting tyrants, progenitors of the European psychosis, raping and despoiling their women, men, and their children in a depraved orgy of sexual misappropriation? How do we come to terms with the madness of a psychosis that demands that these people of color survive in the lunatic environment of racism, prejudice, bigotry, discrimination, intolerance, microaggression, racial profiling, name-calling, bullying and racial baiting, where their social power is subordinated and their daily existence is bombarded by hate crimes, murder, lynching, mass shootings, terrorism, torture, and abuse?

These questions have been systematically and undeniably answered by detailed scholarship of the descendants of Africans enslaved in the New World. The work of Douglas Hall [2] and Orlando Patterson [3] leads the scholarship of the Jamaican Caribbean experience. Did the ruthless eradication of the languages of Africans enslaved in the New World, as Marlene Norbese Philip suggests [4], obliterate the linguistic resources necessary to create, control or even understand the products of their own imagination? Rex Nettleford anticipated this assertion 17 years before Philip, suggesting that in the absence of a strongly preserved cultural memory and in the wake of the deliberate uprooting of ancestral institutions by the slave system, the African slave was to become the nearest thing to a *tabula rasa* on which the new vocabulary of Creole existence could be written [5]. Of all those who were brought to the plantation societies of the New World, it is the descendants of enslaved Africans who have become the prime agents of the creativity driving all the experiments in new ways of living. Nettleford further suggested that the New World descendant is Europe's melody and Africa's rhythm, at once the dissonance and the harmony of both. He thinks 'him pickney (children) white' while fully knowing that everyone else knows that he is Black [5]. Nettleford's observations were underscored in an article, titled 'Roast Breadfruit Psychosis', that I co-authored in 1999 with Trinidadian Gerard Hutchinson on disturbed racial identification in African Caribbeans [6].

Nettleford reminds us that the Black Caribbean still finds himself fighting for recognition and status more than a century after legal emancipation, and that his own racial identity coincides with his society's fight for independence not only from Governors, Colonial Secretaries, and Chief Justices, but from the whole matrix of metropolitan customs, prejudices, and preferences which are proving irrelevant or may be stifling of creativity in his new society. Hugh Hodges describes the Jamaican collective experience that finds articulation in:

> the rituals of Kumina, Pocomania, Revivalism, and other Jamaican religions; in Marcus Garvey's Universal Negro Improvement Association; in corn husking competitions and grounds clearings; in Jonkonoo, in Rasta groundings, and in the dance hall. Not coincidentally, all these communal experiences involve song—hymns, chants, work songs, ring tunes, mentos, ska and reggae songs. Jamaican poetry, simply by virtue of being closer to song than fiction, is closer to those communal experiences than fiction can ever be. Consequently poetry is less likely to reflect a marooned consciousness than a Maroon consciousness, a consciousness of being part of a community which however exiled and embattled, has the resources it needs to survive and take root. The African experience was not of being marooned but of being exiled…Revival singers speak of themselves as the Israelites, captive in Egypt or Babylon. Rastafarian songs look forward to a time when all Jah's children will march forward to Zion [7].

Hodges insists that Jamaican poetry and music tell a long story of oppression and defiance, independence and betrayal, which is often unavailable to the reader or the listener. If we are going to talk about Jamaican poetry, we must learn to speak, or at least understand, the Jamaican language. It is in this context that therapeutic use of the concept *collective poetry making* as a seminal component of the psychological analytic and therapeutic method embedded in *psychohistoriographic cultural therapy* has been described by tracing the essence of its therapeutic and transforming mode, and to chronicle its role internationally over the past fifty years [8].

Poetry is, according to the definition provided by Merriam-Webster, a form of literature that uses the expression of feelings and ideas given intensity by the use of distinctive style and rhythm that formulates a concentrated imaginative awareness of experience in language chosen and arranged to create a specific emotional response through meaning, sound, and rhythm; the art of rhythmical composition, written or spoken, for exciting pleasure by beautiful imaginative or elevated thoughts—a literary work in metrical form [9]. William Wordsworth defined poetry as 'the spontaneous overflow of feelings; it takes its origin from emotion recollected in tranquillity…' [10]. Raab suggests that 'a poem has a distinct rhythm. Poetry can also share transformative moments or revelations. Regardless of the type of poem, poetry uses an economy of words; therefore, every word is important. The more specific the poem, the better it is. The best poetry inspires readers to reflect, dream, reminisce, observe, and fantasize. Poems are written in fragments, and each line should have a singular image and feeling' [11].

The Poiesis of Psychohistoriographic Cultural Therapy

Poiesis (from Ancient Greek: ποίησις) is 'the activity in which a person brings something into being that did not exist before' [12]. The term 'cultural poiesis' was coined by Kathleen Stewart as 'an effort (a) to somehow record the state of emergence that animates things cultural and (b) to track some of the effects of this state of things—the proliferation of everyday practices that arise in the effort to know what is happening or to be part of it, for instance, or the haunting or exciting presence of traces, remainders, and excesses uncaptured by claimed meanings' [13].

The concept of the collective poem is a seminal component of the psychological analytic and therapeutic method *psychohistoriographic cultural therapy* (PCT) which was pioneered in Jamaica in 1977 and which has been used in diverse cultures for mental health therapy and psychosociological change. A critical component of the methodology and therapeutic use of PCT includes the incorporation of all forms of *poetry making* embedded in the PCT technique. By tracing the origin of the therapeutic and transforming mode of PCT, and to chronicle its essence in this study of *Madnificent Irations* in which the process has been used for postcolonial institutional transformation over the past fifty years this article will link the poiesis of PCT with the concept of 'word, sound and power', which is an essential ingredient of Rastafari ritual.

Operational Components of PCT

Led by a trained/experienced cultural therapist, the components of the PCT model consist of *circling*, *centering*, *culturing*, *cognitive catalysis*, and *capacity building*. Starting with cultural circles within large groups of participants, *circling* is a method derived from the kgotla—a large group circular communication system in existence from the very foundation of African society [14]. The participants in the PCT process are invited to 'find their center' by exposure to *centering*—a series of collective mindfulness callisthenic and breathing exercises [15]. Dialectical conversation aids the psychohistoriographic analysis. This type of conversation resembles the dialogism [16], the dialogic cultural circles [17], group ethnography [18] in small or large groups, and the reasoning sessions of Rastafari where dialectical ethnographic discussions become a fundamental requirement for the PCT process. Dialogism is an ongoing chain or network of statements and responses, in which new statements presuppose earlier statements and anticipate future responses. Facilitated by a skilled cultural therapist, dialogism helps the group to delve deeply into their collective truths.

Followed by the process of *culturing* ('art to define values and mission' [19]) using a series of musical, spoken word, and physical dance exercises, the group is invited to explore the historicity of their culture by capturing the ideas, customs, and social behavior of the group using psychohistoriographic analysis [20]. This facilitates *cognitive catalysis* or embodied cognition [21], explored by demanding that each individual create and express a thought and express it to the group in word and action. The specific modality of PCT, collective poetry making is a product of embodied cognition—the perception of the mutual influence of mind and body [22]—of the group reasoning process. Active individual cognition connected to the group dialectic anecdotal historicity and to the emerging group dynamics is the essence of PCT large group psychotherapy. As the reasoning progresses, the PCT analyst 'captures' words and phrases from different persons in the group as they emerge and records them openly on a flipchart, thus tapping each individual's 'inner stream of consciousness' in the engagement of the dialogic discourse with others. The PCT analyst must have experience in group dynamics and group process. PCT therapists tend to initiate the group process, usually by helping to determine the dialectical polarities of the group reasoning, as opposed to conventional psychodynamic therapists who tend to follow the group process rather than initiate it. Initially and throughout, the leader uses real authority in establishing viable therapeutic boundaries and mechanisms. The role of leader inevitably invites transference reactions, where leaders often evoke extremely powerful feelings from their subordinates, not infrequently negative; it requires considerable perseverance, courage, tolerance of uncertainty, and skill.

The PCT leader uses and channels the group dynamics in the *poetry making* and *poem capture*. A secondary therapist is often valuable in this process for capturing the concentrated imaginative awareness of the discussed experiences and emotions, paying strict attention to double meanings, sound and metric rhythm of the spoken word within the group reasoning. This is often carried out by instructing the secondary therapist to document on a flipchart the mimesis and word utterance as the 'PCT reasoning' progresses. Alternatively, this poem making can be carried out alone by the skilled individual PCT therapist without the help of a secondary therapist. The group is encouraged to read the poem aloud as the creation develops, so that it develops insight about the shape and direction of the poetic formation. The group collectively decides when the poem is completed, and collectively reads it aloud and makes selective edits to the shape the style and the poetic meter. As each poem is completed the group can decide on the creation of new poems designated by the dialogic reasoning and initiate the further development into a script for a pageant or play.

The embodiment of *cognitive catalysis* is reflected in Gestalt therapy, a client-centered approach to psychotherapy which often uses role playing to aid the resolution of past conflicts [23]. The final stages of PCT facilitate the dramaturgic production [24] and performance of the PCT-created collective poems, songs, dances, skits/plays [25] and constitutes the basis of *capacity building*. Using the thematic framework from the psychohistoriogram arising from the analysis as a skeleton, the collective and individual poetry and anecdotes/stories can be arranged into a collectively written script, as a play, a pageant, or a song. This may be followed by formal or informal 'recitations' of the poem, whereby the participants perform or dramatize it as a play or pageant in front of a selected audience. Oral poetry that is composed and performed spontaneously in the form of 'dub poetry' spoken over drum or reggae rhythms also becomes a seminal part of the process. The process is usually concluded by each participant being asked to verbally present a judgment of the seminar, and then by a written questionnaire. The results of both oral and written evaluations can be analyzed using qualitative research methods of data collection and analysis; these include observing, documenting and interpreting attributes, patterns, characteristics and meanings of specific, contextual or Gestalt features of phenomena.

Rastafari 'Word Sound and Power' and PCT

With the advent of the history being told by psychologists, using the psychological methodological analytical tool developed in Jamaica called psychohistoriography, the concept of cultural therapy has emerged in the 'overstanding' of the history of the Jamaican people. I have previously suggested that the psychohistoriographic analysis exposes the resilience of the enslaved African people through the emergence of Ethiopianism, which stoutly resisted the ravages of European colonization [26]. The premise is advanced that Ethiopianism has catalyzed a spontaneous irrevocable cultural therapy process providing the basis for worldwide ongoing cultural healing and the liberation of people of color. The nineteenth-century political struggles and Ethiopianism of Paul Bogle and Robert Love drove the emergence of Rastafari and propelled the revolutionary vision of the twentieth century [27].

Many White psychiatrists have suggested that psychotherapy is not appropriate for minority groups because of their supposed lack of 'verbal facility' or the ability to understand and 'work through' their problems in a way that accords with the psychological model. PCT provides standalone insights, stimulating activity that requires the adoption of collective poetry making/writing. This leads to the capture of *psychic centrality* by the collective poem that emerges from the group ethnographic process. This is a concept that has been derived from the PCT process as the sense of psychological containment or organization of diverse individual points of view through creating a historical map of collective experience and is the essence of PCT. Psychic centrality provides a way to explore individual and collective identity [28]. The psychic centrality is the living embodiment of Carl Jung's 'collective unconscious' as an '…idea that has been stamped on the human brain for aeons. That is why it lies ready to hand in the unconscious of every man. Only, certain conditions are needed to cause it to appear…' [29]. A pioneer in psychoanalysis, Jung argued that a major role of psychotherapy is healing of the imagination.

In his book *Poiesis: The Language of Psychology and the Speech of the Soul* (1997) Stephen K. Levine argued that poiesis, the creative act, is also the act by which we affirm our identity and humanity. He opined that not only did psychotherapy reveal the power of the imagination in mental life, but that therapists also slowly became aware that the cure of imaginary disorders could not come from purely rational processes but only through a renovation of the imagination itself. Freud's method of free association, in its encouragement of the fantasy life of the patient, and Jung's concept of active imagination, in its facilitation of a waking state of imaginative potency, showed that a major part of psychotherapy is the healing of the imagination by the imagination. Levine suggested that that the cure for emotional suffering does not come from purely rational processes but through renovation of the imagination. For

Levine, imagination is renovated when it is rid of pathological suffering, that is, fantasies (thought processes) that are stereotypical, compulsive, repetitive, and destructive of self and others. He suggested that this is facilitated by art, which gives a voice to suffering, by expressing the pain and confusion of the disintegration of the self, and, in so doing, enables clients to face themselves without reservation to dance suffering, to paint it or put it into poetic form is to confront it directly and to give oneself up to it. In this expressive moment, Levine suggested, one lets go of attachment to the former security and is willing to face the void. The arts are pathways or methods that take us deeper into ourselves and our experience. As we enter unreservedly into the depth of ourselves, we encounter healing energies and experience the hope of integration. The poesis of poetry, he suggested, is the language of psychology, and concludes that poetry is a tool by which imagination can be laid bare and renovated. However, far too often, he opined, traditional psychotherapy relies solely on the rational processes of the individual to the exclusion of culture, arts, and of the collective. Such tradition is particularly detrimental to 'post-colonial' societies whose cultures have been decimated and collective unconscious stifled by imperialism. A reliance on what is 'rational' from the perspective of a dominant other (the analyst) risks reinforcing the stereotypical thought processes of the dominant culture, which is a further negation of the colonized. Psychohistoriographic cultural therapy addresses these negations and renovates the collective imagination of the colonized, using non-traditional and creative forms of group psychotherapy and social restructuring [30].

Madnificent Irations illustrates and underscores the therapeutic and transformatory power of poetry in politically and emotionally contradictory circumstances. Bakhtin [16] suggested that the use of language is always individual and contextualized and although a word is expressed by an individual, all utterances are the 'product of the interaction of the interlocutors...the product of the whole complex social situation in which it has occurred' (p. 30). 'Dialogic conversation' involves mutual inquiry: an engaged connection of sharing, exploring, crisscrossing, and weaving of ideas, thoughts, opinions, and feelings through which newness and possibility emerge. Responding to Bakhtin, Harlene Anderson asserts that a critical feature of dialog is an interactive two-way process [31]. The collective poetry making process of PCT involves a community with a continued process of cultural identification and 'smadification' [32] effecting change. Suman Fernando described the technique of 'psychohistoriography' and forms of psychotherapy derived from it as effectively challenging traditional Western views about the genesis of 'mental illness' and made the point that the domination of the non-Western world by the West has had a profound effect on the disciplines of psychology and psychiatry. He affirmed that PCT is specifically useful for professionals in the mental health field working with people from Black and other minority ethnic backgrounds [33].

There is a view which dismisses the validity of psychotherapy for Black people, and that race plays a crucial role in the psychotherapeutic process. Some authors, theorists, and researchers have argued that Blacks are not suitable for psychotherapy because of their inherited personality characteristics (e.g., resistance, suspiciousness), their inability to comprehend the nature of psychotherapy (e.g., the verbal self-exploratory process), and the effects of their oppressed status in America and other societies [34]. In addition, White middle-class mental health professionals have typically treated Blacks and other visible racial/ethnic group people as if they were devoid of specific cultures. *Madnificent Irations*, together with the PCT method which emerged from it, has put paid to the Western psychiatric authorities who have proclaimed that Black people are devoid of culture, and established a concrete example of a group psychotherapeutic process with demonstrable outcomes for a tangible group of people of color, in this case, descendants of Africans enslaved in the New World. *Madnificent Irations* demonstrates the powerful influence of Rastafari philosophy and the transformatory role of the PCT process, with a potentially revolutionary effect on people of color worldwide, as I have discussed previously [26].

The emergence of Rastafari was driven by the political struggles of the Jamaican people, with anti colonial champion Marcus Garvey seen as its visionary pioneer [35]. Garvey proposed the systematic antithetical replacement of imposed European cultural values. His vision replaced the European delusion with the African antidote: African religious forms would replace the Judeo-Christian religion. European languages would be replaced by Creole languages and European slave-names would be replaced by African names. New World Africans would re-discover and recover their identity. African art, music, and dance would take preeminence over European art, music, and dance as the predominant cultural form. It was necessary to recreate New World African authority and social systems to replace European authority systems and social systems that had kept Africans enslaved for nearly five hundred years. The metamorphosis would also require New World African Economic orders to replace the dominant European economic systems. Thus, Garvey's message was a profound articulation of *systematic cultural therapy* facilitating transformation of African Diaspora people, thereby countering the imposition of the European-American delusion on people of African origin and people of color. Black people had to find a way to live with their imperialistic aggressors—the European colonizers and slave masters who had imposed a vicious template of social engineering on African people worldwide. I have previously suggested that the emergence of Rastafari catalyzed a spontaneous irrevocable cultural therapy process, providing the basis for a worldwide ongoing cultural healing and the liberation of people of color [26]. The case study of *Madnificent Irations* presented here suggested that this spontaneous cultural therapy revolution catapulted out of psychohistoriographic cultural therapy as a systematized, organized therapeutic antidote against the mental enslavement of European colonialism in the late 1970s reflected in the narratives of the reggae musicians and the psycho-political transformation of Bellevue Hospital.

Bibliography

1. Hickling FW (1985) Poem "Westminster System" (Unpublished).
2. Hall D (1989) *In Miserable Slavery: Thomas Thistlewood in Jamaica 1750–1786*. London: Macmillan.
3. Patterson O (1976) *The Sociology of Slavery: An Analysis of the Origins, Development and Structure of Negro Slave Society in Jamaica*. London: Granada Publishing.
4. Philip MN (1989) *She Tries Her Tongue, Her Silence Softly Breaks*. Middletown, CT: Wesleyan University Press.
5. Nettleford RM (1972) *Identity, Race, and Protest in Jamaica*. New York: William Morrow and Company, Inc., p. 185.
6. Hickling FW, Hutchinson G (1999) Roast Breadfruit Psychosis: Disturbed Racial Identification in African-Caribbeans. *Psychiatric Bulletin, 23*, 132–134.
7. Hodges H (2008) *Soon Come: Jamaican Spirituality, Jamaican Poetics*. Charlottesville: University of Virginia Press, p. 6.
8. Hickling FW, Robertson-Hickling H, Chambers DA (2019, In Press) Collective Poetry Making in the Poesis of Psychohistoriographic Cultural Therapy. *Caribbean Journal of Education*.
9. Merriam-Webster Dictionaries (2013).

10. Wordsworth W (1968) *Lyrical Ballads*, eds. RL Brett and AR Jones. London and New York: Routledge.
11. Raab D (2019) How Poetry Can Heal. *Psychology Today*, April 11.
12. Polkinghorne D (2004) *Practice and the Human Sciences: The Case for a Judgment-Based Practice of Care*. Albany: SUNY Press, p. 115.
13. Stewart K (2005) Cultural Poesis: The Generativity of Emergent Things. *The Sage Handbook of Qualitative Research*, pp. 1027–1042. https://www.sas.upenn.edu/folklore/center/ordinary_affects.pdf.
14. Kgotla—A Public Meeting, Where All Are Allowed to Speak and Where Community Decisions Are Always Arrived at by Consensus (Wikipedia 2019; Your Botswana 2017).
15. Kabat-Zinn J (2003) Mindfulness-Based Interventions in Context: Past, Present, and Future. *Clinical Psychology: Science and Practice*, 10, 144–156.
16. Bakhtin MM (1992) Contemporary Vitalism. Trans. Charles Byrd. In F Burwick, P Douglass (Eds.), *The Crisis in Modernism: Bergson and the Vitalist Controversy*. Cambridge: Cambridge University Press, pp. 76–97.
17. Freire P (1968) *Pedagogy of the Oppressed*. New York: Seabury Press.
18. Geertz C (1973) Toward Interpretive Theory of Culture. In *The Interpretation of Cultures: Selected Essays*. New York: Basic Books, Inc., pp. 3–30.
19. Carnwath JD, Brown AS (2014) Understanding the Value and Impacts of Cultural Experiences: A Literature Review. *Arts Council of England*. https://www.artscouncil.org.uk/publication/understanding-value-and-impacts-cultural-experiences.
20. Hickling (2007) *Psychohistoriography: A Postcolonial Psychoanalytic and Psychotherapeutic Model*. Mona, Jamaica: CARIMENSA Press, University of the West Indies; London: Jessica Kingsley Publishers (2012).
21. Wilson RA, Foglia L (2011) Embodied Cognition. In EN Zalta (Ed.) *The Stanford Encyclopaedia of Philosophy*. https://plato.stanford.edu/archives/fall2011/entries/embodied-cognition/.
22. Randolph PT (2016) Applying Elements of Embodied Cognition to ELL Poetry Read-a-Thons. *CATESOL News, 48*(3).
23. Perls F, Hefferline R, Goodman P (1951) *Gestalt Therapy: Excitement and Growth in the Human Personality*. Goldsboro, ME: Gestalt Journal Press.
24. Jones P (1996) *Drama as Therapy, Theatre as Living*. London and New York: Routledge.
25. Landy RJ (2008) *The Couch and the Stage: Integrating Words and Action in Psychotherapy*. Lanham, MD: Jason Aronson.
26. Hickling FW (2014) Rastafari as an African Diaspora National Liberation Movement. *Jamaica Journal, 35*(1–2), 48–63.
27. Chevannes B (1995) *Rastafari: Roots and Ideology*. New York: Syracuse University Press.

28. Hickling FW, Guzder J, Robertson-Hickling H, Snow S, Kirmayer LJ (2010) Psychic Centrality: Reflections on Two Psychohistoriographic Workshops in Montreal. *Transcultural Psychiatry, 47*, 136.
29. Jung CG (1917) *Collected Works of C. G. Jung, Volume Seven: Two Essays on Analytical Psychology*, eds. H Read, M Fordham, G Adler. Princeton University Press, 1966, p. 109. Downloaded from https://www.holybooks.com/c-g-jung-collected-works-free-pdf/.
30. Levine SK (1997) *Poiesis: The Language of Psychology and the Speech of the Soul.* London: Jessica Kingsley Ltd. Kindle Edition (locations 85–88).
31. Anderson H (2012) Collaborative Relationships and Dialogic Conversations: Ideas for a Relationally Responsive Practice. *Family Process, 51*, 8–24.
32. Scott D, Nettleford RM (June 2006) "To Be Liberated from the Obscurity of Themselves": An Interview with Rex Nettleford. *Small Axe, Number 20*, 10(2), 97–246.
33. Fernando SJ (2013) Book Review: Psychohistoriography: A Post-Colonial Psychoanalytic and Psychotherapeutic Model. *British Journal of Psychiatry, 203*, 77.
34. Carter R (1995) *The Influence of Race and Racial Identity in Psychotherapy: Towards a Racially Inclusive Model.* London and New York: Wiley, p. 48.
35. Lewis R (1987) *Marcus Garvey: Anti-Colonial Champion.* London: Karia Press.

CHAPTER 10

Cultural Therapy and Social Engineering

Let us put aside de differences
That have caused us to divide
And find the common enemy
That keeps Tribe still fighting Tribe. [1]

The theme song '*Step by step*' of *Madnificent Irations* in 1978 laid out unequivocally the message of the painstaking journey that the recovering mentally ill were sending to the people of Jamaica '…*Wey de righteous must stan an de wicked must fall*…' Nearly thirty years later, Jamaica, with a homicide rate of 53/100,000 in 2005, had the third highest rate of lethal violence in the world [2], thereby sending the message that interpersonal violence remained the most significant Jamaican mental health problem. Jamaican society seems extraordinarily tolerant and even accommodating of violence in its various forms. *Madnificent Irations* argued that violence, originally manifested as rebellion against political, economic, and racial exploitation, was turned inward as tribalism and self-destruction, following the adoption of the Westminster system of parliamentary democracy in the 1940s. The lessons of conflict and division in the development of cultural therapy in Bellevue Hospital in 1978, and the destruction of the Garden Theatre and the cultural therapy program at the hospital in 1982 illustrated starkly for us why politics has divided us and continues to divide us in Jamaica and to understand how politics in Jamaica has come to hold such polarized prejudices.

F. W. Hickling, *Decolonization of Psychiatry in Jamaica*,
https://doi.org/10.1007/978-3-030-48489-7_10

An important answer emerges if one carries out a *psychohistoriographic analysis* of how the political parties came into being in this Jamaica. In 1938, there existed a single political party in Jamaica seeking liberation from colonial exploitation; it was called the People's National Party (PNP), with Norman Manley and Alexander Bustamante being founder members and at that time everybody was pulling together against British colonialism. *Madnificent Irations* makes reference to Bustamante's speech made in 1938, which was more radical than any speech I have ever heard or read made by any politician in Jamaica:

> ...It will be bloodshed. There will be bloodshed. I expect everyone in this country to follow. We will let these employers respect us. We will take away their lands and give them to the workers. We shall fight with vengeance, we shall be ruthless with hate. From Kingston to Negril shall be in the fight and if the government says we cannot keep meetings, we will go in the forests, riverside and bush... The niggers of this country shall rise. We do not want to go to war like a timid dog. There will be war. We want revolution in this country and before whites destroy us we will destroy them... [3]

Bustamante was inciting the crowd to join him in tearing down the capitalist system—to destroy all the White people who had colonized our country and to throw them into the sea. The fragments of telegrams from Sir Arthur Richards, the Colonial Governor at the time, to his superiors in the Home Office advised explicitly that the colonial government had to deal definitively with Bustamante. The British dealt with these things all over the world, all the time, by the process of divide and rule. So they put Bustamante in prison for four years, and while he was in prison, they fed him a steady diet of misinformation, such as: '... Manley is taking away your Union, Manley is taking away your people...', feeding on the narcissism of the man in an atmosphere of intense paranoia deliberately inculcated in the sensory deprivation of almost total isolation. By incarcerating him, the colonial government succeeded in splitting the Jamaican revolutionary political movement.

Bustamante had made an agreement in 1938 that while he was in prison Manley would look after his Union on his behalf, and Manley was doing just that. A PNP politician of the time told me some years ago that Manley had made a commitment to Bustamante: '...while you are in prison I will look after your Union, don't worry about it, we will sort it out...'. The British captors, in the meanwhile, whispered in

Bustamante's ear '...Manley taking over your Union, Manley taking over your Union...'. Jamaica Labour Party (JLP) activist and trade unionist Pearnel Charles assured me of his belief that Father Manley was indeed trying to take over Bustamante's trade union base. Whether true or not, in an oppressive environment of isolated incarceration, psychological disinformation was easily sown and nurtured. The British made an agreement with Bustamante to form an opposing political party that would take over the working-class mass movement which he had helped to initiate. The Jamaican people had been effectively split into two political 'tribes', and by 1944, with the granting of universal adult suffrage under a Westminster system of government to the people of Jamaica, the British government had effectively cemented the European hegemony for the remainder of the century, by pitting Blacks against each other in the classic 'divide and rule' strategy of the European colonizer. Willie Lynch's purported formula of *fear, distrust, and envy* had won the day again for the colonizers.

This was the basis of the colonial government's agreement to free Bustamante. Of course he agreed and thus came about the birth of the Jamaica Labour Party, which was a combination now of working-class activists and the plantocracy. By this means the plantocracy was able to retain its hold on power. The next fifty years of political life in Jamaica were to prove beyond a doubt that the European ideology had been effectively ingrained in the psyche of the political life and government of this country, and that its interests no longer needed Europeans to maintain it. In short, tribal party politics in postcolonial countries never serve the interests of the majority of the people, but serve the continued interests of European world domination. Obika Gray chronicles the day and the date and the hour when the violence was introduced in the political landscape—the genesis of Jamaican political violence; Bellevue Hospital featured in this eventful drama [4]. Coming out of our ethnohistorical reasonings at Bellevue Hospital in the 1970s, we discovered from the anecdotes of our staff and patients who were alive at the time that the first political death in Jamaica took place in 1946 during a workers' strike at the hospital. The strike was the prelude to a clash between Bustamante (of the JLP) and Glasspole (of the PNP) on the streets; for the first time in contemporary Jamaica, somebody had been killed by the tribal violence between the two political formations of the 1940s. Alexander Bustamante and Frank Pixley were arrested, tried, and subsequently acquitted of manslaughter arising out of the death of John Nicholas and Clifford Reid of Kingston

[5]. Jamaican political history is replete with instances of social engineering designed to influence popular attitudes and social behavior on a large scale. Governments, media, politicians, and private groups have used social engineering by inciting and repeating social events. Once the social event triggered a successful outcome, it was repeated again and again with the aim of bringing about the desired outcome.

The Need for Social Re-engineering in Jamaica

After independence in 1962, Jamaica seemed urgently in need of psychological rescue programs aimed at combating the social engineering of subservience and psychopathology in its people, spawned by the four hundred years of slavery and colonialism by the European-American psychosis. The question about Jamaica's need for social re-engineering was posed to me during the sitting of the four-man Board of Enquiry established by the Ministry of Health in July 1978 to enquire into the complaints made by the nurses and clerks of Bellevue Hospital against me as Senior Medical Officer (SMO) during the implementation of the cultural therapy and rehabilitation programs at that hospital. Minister of Health Dr. Douglas Manley had appointed the Board of Enquiry to investigate a complaint made to the Ministry on May 30 by the nurses, represented by the Jamaica Union of Public Officers and Public Employees (JUPOPE) and the Nurses Association of Jamaica (NAJ) that they were being constantly abused by the SMO and gangs of people who invaded the hospital, as well as members of the auxiliary staff. The Board members were: Mr. David Muirhead QC, chairman; Dr. Mary Seivwright, representing the NAJ; Dr. Vernon O. Lindo, representing the Medical Association of Jamaica; and Mr. Leslie Wynter, representing JUPOPE [6].

During the enquiry, the Board assessed the evidence that the SMO was establishing a therapeutic community rehabilitation process through the cultural therapy program that was being developed to transform the 100-year custodial incarceration program of 'custodial care', established by the British colonial government in 1862. The Board members asked for me to provide evidence as to whether I had the training and expertise to establish such social engineering programs. I had to establish that I had been trained in social engineering and rehabilitation processes by famous international experts such as Professor Eugene Brody of the University of Maryland, and Professor Morris Carstairs and Dr.

Jack Affleck of the University of Edinburgh, and that I had received practical experience of these processes at the therapeutic community program at Dingleton Hospital in Scotland that had been established by the father of modern therapeutic community principles, Dr. Maxwell Jones. The Board agreed that the rehabilitation cultural therapy programs that I was establishing were sound, appropriate, and legitimate. The Board dispatched me to resume my work and instructed the confrontational nurses and administrators to work with the program.

The Wikipedia entry for social engineering describes it as a discipline in social science that 'refers to efforts to influence popular attitudes and social behaviors on a large scale, whether by governments, media, or private groups' [7]. My doctoral thesis for the degree of Doctor of Medicine (Psychiatry) supervised by one of the fathers of African psychiatry from the University of Lagos, Nigeria, Professor Tolani Asuni, was a scientific study of the social engineering pilot that I had established at Bellevue Hospital in 1974 [8]. It is not surprising therefore that as soon as I became Professor of Psychiatry at the University of the West Indies (UWI) in 2000, and in keeping with the UWI Strategic Objectives developed in 2000, I pioneered the creation of a primary prevention mental health organization, the Caribbean Institute of Mental Health and Substance Abuse (CARIMENSA) in 2005. Based on the pioneering work of *Madnificent Irations* and the creation of the cultural therapy model in the mental hospital in 1978, the central tenet of this institute was and is the promulgation of primary prevention in the area of mental health, focusing on the development of *psychohistoriographic cultural therapy* and the creation of centers for cultural therapy for social engineering in the Caribbean. The establishment of a Masters of Science in Cultural Therapy was a seminal creation of the UWI in 2008 [9]. The CARIMENSA vision is to generate and facilitate the implementation of creative and innovative strategies which promote mental wellness, wealth creation, and productivity at the individual and community levels. The MSc in Cultural Therapy is the training ground which will equip individuals with the knowledge and skills needed to move this vision into action. The program has been designed to develop students' competence in cultural therapy as well as in a number of other areas in health, research, education, the arts, and the social sciences. The aim is for graduates to be well-rounded persons capable of driving the positive changes that are required in many areas of society. In 2013, Ms. Kathi Thomas was the first graduate of this novel program [10]. Her pioneering work in this area has led her in helping to develop a classical music orchestra containing 120 inner-city adolescent boys in Kingston.

Media Representation Research and Psychological Deinstitutionalization

In 2008, Dr. Rob Whitley of McGill University and I co-authored a paper on media representations of psychiatric de-institutionalization in Jamaica by collecting and analyzing all stories published by Jamaica's principal broadsheet *The Daily Gleaner* between January 2003 and March 2005 related to psychiatric de-institutionalization [11]. All of the 21 relevant articles flagged up by the search were positive and enlightened in orientation. Our research noted three overlapping processes within the articles that attempted to allay supposed fears and concerns—the strategic use of expert informants; appeals to reason by quoting international trends and statistics; and scientific education of the general public in lay language. We posited that these rhetorical processes are component parts of a wider phenomenon we labeled 'psychiatric de-institutionalization'.

Between 1970 and 2011 2261 articles on mental illness and mental health appeared in the five major newspapers: *The Daily Gleaner* (53%), *The Jamaica Star* (19%), *Daily News* (13%), *Jamaica Observer* (7.9%), and *Jamaica Herald* (5%). This represented an average of 5 articles per month with an annual range from a maximum of 128 in 1970 to a minimum of 24 in 1983. The vast majority (98%) of these newspaper reports were about social engineering issues surrounding mental health in Jamaica, with 34% on mental health education, 32% on the development of community mental health services, and 32% on political and ideological debate on mental health challenges. The analysis of this data is ongoing, but the important initial finding is an attitudinal trend that shifted from negative reports of homicide, suicide, and crime by the mentally ill in the years between 1970 and 1980 to positive and enlightened articles published decades later in the years between 2000 and 2010, which related mainly to the positive effects of community mental health. The critical finding of this analysis was the shift from negative to positive reporting of mental health issues by the broadsheet newspapers in 404 articles (an average of 67 per year) between 1977 and 1982.

What is significant is that this was the period of the social re-engineering of Bellevue Hospital with the launch of *Madnificent Irations*, the birth of cultural therapy, and the deliberate objective of the rehabilitation of the mentally ill, using cultural therapy and the release from custodial incarceration [12]. Independence from British colonialism has catalyzed Jamaica to provide liberating, humanizing, efficacious, cost-effective, and culturally appropriate approaches to treating mental illness by integrating mental health into all levels of the health system including general hospitals, primary care, and the community to provide accessible, affordable mental health care for the population. Creative and visionary leadership of indigenous mental health practitioners over 50 years has fostered an in-tandem combination of two innovative strategies: *cultural therapy* for the gradual deinstitutionalization of the mental hospital; the *integration* of psychiatry with the public health system by treating mental illness in the community. The goals were the abolition of custodial care facilities for the mentally ill, geographic catchmenting of mental health services island wide, development of culturally appropriate methods of treating mental illness, and reduction in stigma toward the mentally ill in the community. The final goal was the establishment of community social re-engineering strategies, including cultural therapy, for children and adults.

This extraordinary mental health social re-engineering process has resulted in the dramatic reduction of the size of the psychiatric mental hospital from 110 to 40 acres; bed reduction from 3100 in 1960 to 550 in 2017. Since 1974, the Community Mental Health Service (CMHS) has merged with primary and secondary health care delivery island wide, with 3 in 4 psychiatric hospital admissions made to general hospitals and 60,000 people with severe enduring mental illness being successfully treated in 105 clinics located in parish communities across the island. Few countries in the developed or developing world can boast that persons with acute severe mental illness can receive satisfactory treatment within 24 hours anywhere in the country. There have been several intentional and unintentional consequences. Recent studies have demonstrated a reduction of stigma toward mental illness. Training psychiatrists and other mental health professionals in Jamaica have reversed the mental health professional brain drain. Significant reduction of the costs of managing acute and severe enduring mental illness has been another result. Early integration of mental health professionals into clinical and administrative health facilities in the country has resulted in the assessment and treatment of most psychiatric illnesses by medical practitioners and at general hospitals. This has catalyzed the development and growth of research publications and the promotion of positive approaches to mental health.

The most significant initial obstacle to the process was resistance from clinicians and administrators at every level of practice. Dismantling the administrative and clinical organization of the custodial mental hospital remains the greatest hurdle. The overarching unintended consequence of this psychiatric metamorphosis was the *gradual assimilation* of psychiatry into general medicine. The extremely successful Jamaican cultural therapy application for dysfunctional and underperforming children called *Dream-A-World Cultural Therapy* won the 'Turning the World Upside Down' competition in London in 2013 for the most successful mental health innovation from low- and middle-income countries, which could be effectively applied to major health challenges faced by high-income countries. Organized in collaboration with MIND, the Centre for Global Mental Health, NYU's Program in Global Mental Health, the Institute for Health Improvement, the London School of Hygiene and Tropical Medicine and Maudsley International, the Mental Health Challenge attracted 34 entries worldwide. Jane McGrath in her blog [13] said: 'I wanted then to share with you The Dream-A-World Cultural Therapy intervention for promoting resilience in High Risk Primary School Children in Jamaica. It was our hands down winner.' She described the process where 30 children with a history of difficult behavior and school failure were asked to imagine (dream) a new world on another planet, name it and conceive its inhabitants, decide what to take or eliminate from their known world to this new one, how they would look, and what role they would play in governing the new world. They then worked with artists for 30 months, learning how to play musical instruments and compose songs, poems, and dances about their new world. Literacy and numeracy sessions were included, as were field trips. The program proved so successful that all 30 children from the 'proof of concept' pilot project passed the Grade Six Achievement Test and entered accredited high schools in Jamaica. McGrath asserted that the real winner should be the mental health community, with an influx of new ideas, successful models of innovative care, and an emphasis throughout on engaging service users, their families, carers, and communities from the start. The *Dream-A-World Cultural Therapy* project has been successfully replicated for 100 inner-city children in Kingston in a 'scale-up' project funded by Grand Challenges Canada in 2013. So successful has this project been that Jamaica's Ministry of Education launched a similar transformatory project in which the *Dream-A-World Cultural Therapy* program morphed into the *Dream-A-World Cultural Resiliency* for 35 poorly performing primary schools in eastern Jamaica [14] in 2014, with CARIMENSA looking to implement a transition to scale project for the 1000 primary schools in Jamaica over a 3-year period. So far, this program has been implemented in 87 primary schools in eastern Jamaica, providing therapeutic transformation for nearly 2000 8-year-olds who had previously been assessed as behaviorally dysfunctional and academically challenged [15].

Taking Community Engagement Cultural Therapy to Kingston's Inner City

Based on the cultural therapy model generated by the development of *Madnificent Irations* and the Garden Theatre at Bellevue Hospital in 1978, community engagement cultural therapy was implemented successfully in the Kingston inner-city garrison community of Seaview Gardens in 2013. Funded by a grant from Grand Challenges Canada to CARIMENSA, the project was developed in collaboration with the Community Mental Health Services of the Jamaican Ministry of Health and Public Mental Health Services. The question was posed as to whether the Garden Theatre model could be successfully replicated to reduce violence and generate mental health and vocational entrepreneurship in a poverty-stricken, violence-ridden garrison community in inner-city Kingston.

Most instances of lethal violence in Jamaica occur in these communities in the Kingston Metropolitan Region. They are rigidly controlled by a socio-political system that engenders pathological dependency, which fuels urban violence in its various forms, and are socially isolated through violence and stigmatization, with an enforced power structure controlled by the garrison area leaders or 'dons', who prevent self-determination. The development of the garrison community in Jamaica is a unique postcolonial feature of the Jamaican political system [16]. Jamaican political economist Dr. George Beckford in his seminal polemic *Persistent Poverty* [17] described postcolonial plantation economies as having provided systematic opportunities for the suppression of the majority, and to ensure the maintenance of a large unskilled labor force for the benefit of the privileged few. The ability of the garrison communities to provide outreach work for their inhabitants greatly enhances their significance. The bipolar homogenization of political expression that comes with the development of garrisons has had an important psychological impact on Jamaican politics. The terrorism associated with the garrison process breeds a deep fear of armed enforcers and their potential for lethal violence. Beckford used the *total institution* model of Dr. Erving Goffman to describe the development of the institution of *plantation society* during slavery. The concept of the garrison presents itself ideologically as a representation of the total institution in the communities of the lower socioeconomic areas. These communities are rigidly controlled by a socio-political system that engenders pathological dependency and fuels urban violence in its various forms. The dons control the distribution of basic goods; they also assign roles and responsibilities for each individual, deciding, for example, who gets to go to work.

As a rule, a community seeks to foster a sense of personal responsibility among its patients. This can be paralleled to the concept of *milieu therapy*, in which patients are encouraged to take personal responsibility for themselves and others and the interaction between staff and patients is no longer dictatorial as in the asylum but instead democratic and resulting in consensus building. This forms the core of the therapeutic community model, which uses empowerment and positive social restructuring as described by Maxwell Jones to negate institutionalization in the mental hospital. As Jones noted, the democratic egalitarian social structure of a therapeutic community threatened the authority of an established hierarchical hospital system. The Jamaican community engagement model of mental health, which uses cultural therapy as a foundation tool, is constructed on the principles of empowerment and collaborative investment. By engaging the innate cultural agency of the community, it may achieve for the garrison communities what it did for the asylum.

Performance centers are spaces where community cultural development can take place. Based on the Jamaican cultural experience, the most basic facility for such activities is a tent and a sports playing field. Through careful planning and community engagement, a wide variety of cultural and sporting activities can be established through which the creative energies of the community are channeled. These activities will constitute the nidus of sustainable economic development of the community, while audio- and videotapes record the development of job creation processes around which newly formed creative industries can flourish.

The Social Re-engineering Coda

Cultural therapy is so powerful that the existing political system actively engages in its destruction. The destruction takes different forms, including politics, 'red eye and bad mind' [18], the presence of gunmen, theft and murder; it can be instigated by the community itself. There is no doubt that the Caribbean people are suffering psychologically as a result of the high levels of violence in the region. Action is required at all levels, including education, continued research, strengthening social cohesion, and the provision of social support and psychological services for those directly affected. The active participation of young people in their communities' and nation's development must be encouraged. They need to be allowed to voice their opinions on issues that affect them. We need to inform and educate the youth on their rights and responsibilities versus power and powerlessness. These ideas should be integrated into school curricula at all levels and into community-based programs with child-friendly definitions and materials. We must tap into the strength of young people to help in reduction of violence in the schools. Finally, we need to empower and allow young people to contribute to developing the solutions. It is also important to explore the possibility of strengthening spiritual bases as a means of preventing violent behavior and building resilience in our youth. The use of community engagement cultural therapy initiatives described above is posited as providing unique signifiers for the transformation of the rising levels of intentional and interpersonal violence, rape and youth crime, and the strengthening of creative cultural and economic activities leading eventually to increased levels of education and employment, especially for the youth. We will negate the social engineering of slavery and colonialism. As Bob Marley sang in 'Redemption Song', from his album *Uprising*: '*...emancipate yourselves from mental slavery; none but ourselves can free our minds...*' [19]. The sociodrama *Madnificent Irations* launched in 1978 at the Bellevue Hospital heralded the birth of psychohistoriographic cultural therapy as a social re-engineering blueprint for emancipating ourselves from mental slavery. '*... Step by step we goin to the Golden Gate... Wey de righteous must stan an de wicked must fall... Only the pure will answer to the call...*'.

My poem *Westminster System*, used as chapter epigraphs for this book, reflects the nature of the postcolonial Westminster system imposed on and experienced by descendants of Africans enslaved in the New World. It suggests a blueprint for our release from the institution of British colonial governance that still entraps us in the Caribbean and in many other countries of the world and demands an immediate solution to the 'divide and rule' policy of British colonialism:

The system left by Westminster
has one intrinsic flaw
It forces us to divide and fight sisters
and brothers with tooth and nail and claw.

Why do we think Westminster's system
Left by Limey as he withdrew
Will really solve our problems
For our ship and all its crew?

He left Elizabeth the Monarch
Sitting smiling on her throne
To overlook our business
While starving Black man groan.

Know that it is the same Westminster
That rules our little nation
Decimated Black man's culture
By building the plantation.

So how are we to expect
a system which protects
The rights of private property
To treat Black man with respect?

Him throw de crumbs gi we again
'Come on Blackie, take the reins'
while him still own all de factory
An de lan an sugar canes.

Let us waken from de slumber
Of de anaesthetic gas
Which has kept us in de ghettos
Of de men's mental morass.

For is him create Westminster
That keeps us still enslaved
To the coat tail of him dunza
An to an image which he made.

Mek we bruck out of de shackles
That still keeps our minds enslaved
Like Procrustes an fe him long bed
Who stretched each man from toe to head.

Let us put aside de differences
That have caused us to divide
And find the common enemy
That keeps Tribe still fighting Tribe.

Bibliography

1. Hickling FW (1985) Poem “Westminster System” (Unpublished).
2. Krause K, Muggah R, Gilgen E (2011) *Global Burden of Armed Violence.* Cambridge: Cambridge University Press.
3. Richards A (1940) Telegram to Secretary of State for the Colonies from Governor of Jamaica—Extract: C.O. 137 840/68511/229 8788 d/d 13/'9/'40.
4. Gray O (2004) *Demeaned but Empowered: the Social Power of the Urban Poor in Jamaica.* Kingston: University of the West Indies Press.
5. *Daily Gleaner* (1946) Bustamante, Pixley Charged with Manslaughter. Kingston, April 12, p. 1.
6. *Sunday Gleaner* (1978) At Bellevue…Nurses Threaten Strike Action. Kingston, July 30, p. 3.
7. Wikipedia, Entry for ‘Social engineering (political science)’. https://en.wikipedia.org/wiki/Social_engineering_(political_science).
8. Hickling FW (1975) *The Establishment of a Rehabilitation Service at Bellevue Mental Hospital, Jamaica, and an Analysis of the First Six Months of That Service.* Degree of Doctor of Medicine (Psychiatry), University of the West Indies.
9. Gibson RC, Mathies BK, Hickling FW (2007) CARIMENSA’s Masters’ Degree in Cultural Therapy. In FW Hickling (Ed.), *Dream a World—CARIMENSA and the Development of Cultural Therapy in Jamaica.* Kingston, Jamaica: CARIMENSA.
10. Thomas KR (2013) *Enhancing Social Skills and Improving Self Esteem in Adolescent Males Through a Cultural Therapy Intervention.* Dissertation for the Masters of Science in Cultural Therapy of the University of the West Indies.

11. Whitley R, Hickling FW (2007) Open Papers, Open Minds? Media Representations of Psychiatric De-institutionalization in Jamaica. *Transcultural Psychiatry, 44*, 659–671. https://doi.org/10.1177/1363461507083903.
12. Littlewood R, Lipsedge M (1989) *Aliens and Alienists: Ethnic Minorities and Psychiatry*. London: Unwin Hyman.
13. McGrath J (2014) In The Dragons Den Turning The World Upside Down? http://www.patientpublicinvolvement.com/in-the-dragons-den-turning-the-world-upside-down-by-jane-mcgrath/.
14. *Jamaica Observer* (2014) 'Dream a World Project to Be Expanded to 35 Primary Schools'. Tuesday, January 6. http://www.jamaicaobserver.com/news/-Dream-A-World-Project--to-be-expanded-to-35-primary-schools_17607305.
15. Hickling FW, Walcott GO (2019) The Jamaican LMIC Challenge to the Biopsychosocial Global Mental Health Model of Western Psychiatry. In S Okpaku (Ed.), *Innovations in Global Mental Health*. Cham: Springer Nature Switzerland AG.
16. Figueroa M, Sives A (2002) Homogenous Voting, Electoral Manipulation and the 'Garrison' Process in Post-Independence Jamaica. *Commonwealth & Comparative Politics, 40*(1), 81–108.
17. Beckford G (1972) *Persistent Poverty: Underdevelopment in Plantation Economies of the Third World*. New York: Oxford University Press.
18. Hickling FW, James C (2008) Traditional Mental Health Practices in Jamaica: On the Phenomenology of Red Eye, Bad Mind and Obeah (Chapter 15). In FW Hickling, BM Matthies, KA Morgan, RC Gibson (Eds.), *Perspectives in Caribbean Psychology*. Kingston: CARIMENSA Press, University of the West Indies, Mona.
19. Bob Marley and The Wailers (1979) "Redemption Song" from the album *Uprising*, produced by Chris Blackwell for Island Records.

Appendix

Madnificent Irations

A Sociodrama Poem

by

Frederick W. Hickling

Dramatis Personae

Madman narrator 1 (mm1)
Madman narrator 2 (mm2)
Madman narrator 3 (mm3)

Bedward
Busha (overseer) 1
Busha 2
Carmen: female patient
Doctor
Female attendant
Gentleman
Judge/Governor
Lawyer 1
Lawyer 2
Male nurse 1
Male nurse 2

F. W. Hickling, *Decolonization of Psychiatry in Jamaica*, https://doi.org/10.1007/978-3-030-48489-7

Male patient
Mr Ready: male attendant
Nurse
Nursing sister
Policeman 1
Policeman 2
Senior Medical Officer (SMO)

Chorus

ACT I

mm1
This is the story of a tribe of proud man
Strong brave man, peaceful, upful man
wid powerful mind and forward spiritual
Uprooted from him fatherland
of him crosses and him worries
an him trial and tribulation
in a new land of Babylon

mm2
But our story has a special find
it deals with spaces of the mind
hitherto regarded mad
But to us, a discovery glad
The fitting place to make a discovery
of that nature in a madhouse
This is a madhouse
That is what we are told
That is what we are called
You tells us that everyday
So we a go ina we headcup
To find out what dis ting really mean

mm1
Is a true story doah
An the story stilla go on
Now we goin have to introduce you
to the players of this strange drama,
an den go ina de story, Iya

mm2
Now, I am a mad man
we are sitting in a mad house
That is what uno call it
Right
No, a mental hospital
Uno dress it up

Male patient
Listen doc, I'm not no fucking mad man
I'm sane doc, I'm sane
I just want to come outa dis place doc
give me my discharge nuh doc
give me my discharge
I want to go home you know doc

	write up I discharge nuh doc write up I discharge me doc me, me doc me see me here, see me here
Doctor	All right all right man, take it easy Take it easy and nurse will look after you Nurse, please look after this young man Nurse this one is getting maniacal Give him shock treatment and sodium amytal grains seven and a half be very careful with him nurse, he's dangerous
mm2	This is the story about a man peaceful upful man, and powerful mind and forward spiritual Uprooted from him fatherland of him crosses and him worries an him trial and tribulation In a new land of Babylon
mm1	So you don't believe it That scene I and I just seen is a true reflection of the treatment scene, seen and in case you might have a doubt mek I show you what I talkin bout
Carmen	Hey you is me fader, is you is me fader you look like mi fader, him tall an handsome an him have tall straight hair, an him white no you can't be mi fader, you too black maybe you is mi husban you black enough to be mi husban you just fuck mi an gi mi nuff nuff pickney den walk off an leave me fuck off, you is a nasty dutty naaga dawg
Nursing sister	Hush Hush Carmen, don't distress yourself leave Mr. Thomas alone, you are not well today dear come and take your tablets
Carmen	You can fuck off wid yu tablets Sister Mi nah tek no more tablets all me want is me husban Who gawn wid the nasty dutty naaga gal All me a do is a tek dis yah pill an tek dat de pill Uno juk juk up mi batty, till it come like pin cushion don't bodder give me no fuckin needle
Nursing sister	Nurse, go give Carmen her medicine come now dear don't give any trouble now Mr. Ready go and help nurse give Carmen her medicine Come on dear don't give any trouble now come and take your tablets

Carmen — You no hear sey me no want none a yu rass tablets
Fuck off and stuff dem in yu nunny
Yu face favour like you want man
Mi no want no injection
Mi no want no ECT
Yu just fry up man brains
let me go, let me go
Dread Lion, ah who you a call mad man
Dread Lion, ah who you a call mad man
Call me man but no call mi mad man
Call mi man but no call mi mad man
Call mi man one man cannot name mad and man
Mad man
Yu better call yu puppa so
Mad man
Yu better call yu mumma so
Mad man
Yu better call yu bredda so
Mad man
Yu better call yu sister so
Mad man
Call me man
but no call me mad man
Dread Lion
call me man
but no call me mad man
Dread Lion

mm1 — These are some more of that tribe of proud man
More players you might say of our little madhouse drama
Those little factual fantasies we just witnessed
were mumma and puppa of the said tribe
but with the one root
you will hear dat dirts again and again ina dis ya sinting
Dread Lion, call me man but no call me mad
Mad man

mm2 — Now this tribe had come from a land far distant
Ten thousand miles across the sea
But it wasn't like we did come on a excursion trip
You know, like you pay yu three hundred dollars an gone
on a round trip cruise on the Starward to Miami and the Bahamas
Dem did come ina boat hold, like cargo
like uno know, ten thousand case a sardine, five thousand
tin a bully beef, fifteen thousand pound of salt pork

Chorus — Five thousand naaga man
Three thousand naaga woman
and fifteen hundred black pickney

mm1 — Oh, and one thousand pounds
of salt

mm2 Yes papa, is Africa dem man did come from
on a white man slave ship
and you know how dem days did stay
How them treated the niggers
guilty conscience, guilt and shame
Some have, but others none
gi dem half a chance
an dem would do it all again
mm1 Den de apologists
Sey dat we mustn't talk
bout slavery, bout Africa
Cause it done happen already
But a fi we history, and I an I puppa
Sey I fi speak de trut and
speak it ever cost it what it will
mm2 So I man will talk
of Africa and I bondage
and downpression still, you know
a just dat, cause it no change
Du muriah mama, Du muriah mama
Du muriah mama, Du muriah oh
Beg you one piece of con-di, Beg you one piece of con-di
Beg you one piece of con-di, Du muriah oh
Tomorrow when dem gawn de, Tomorrow when dem gawn de
Tomorrow when dem gawn de
Badaration de pon yu
mm1 Dem flog we dem beat we
dem tek starvation lik we
dem run we down
an juk me wid long gun
only to mek dem money
while I & I labour in the sun
mm2 Well I expect dat I man did go-awn bad
Mek noise and cuss badwud
and fight off de white soldier dem
But you woulda do de same
if man was a sun you out ina hot sun all day, an drop dutty
lick ina you rass back like you was some animal
Some beast of burden
come to fatten backra massa table
Dem nuh even treat dem dawg dat way
Yu nuh see how dem tie ribbon
under dem dawg neck, and bathe dem
and brush dem like dem a pickney
Well ah not even so dem did treat I & I man
Dem treat I like a beast of burden

	Flog I an chain I and pen I up.
mm1	Proud tribe of Africa, sold to slaving
	dying on the middle passage toiling on the plantation
	Strip I and I of I culture
	I man fight, I man preserve I culture
	White man slavery continues
	I and I fight back, remember Cudjoe
	Dem Baldhead decide to emancipate we
	Slavery was too expensive to run
	Black people fight back too hard
	Free dem but still downpress dem
	Baldhead hold all de money
	Made of the sweat of I an I labour
	Baldhead hold all de land
	Stolen from I an I father hand
mm2	Don't bodder think sey
	dem free we cause dem love we
	I man fight back and struggle
	And is dem have fe pay fe it
mm2	And even though Baldhead now didn't own I
	him still control I
	For ah him control de dunny and own all de lan
	Up till dat time madness did not exist
	in relation to the black man
	he was just a slave
Busha 1	Slaves don't get mad, you crazy
	who ever heard of a mad slave
Busha 2	Ha, we would just have to exterminate him
	like a mad dog
Chorus	Mad dog
	Fire, fire, fire, fire fall on me
	Fire, fire, fire, fire fall on me
	On the day of Pentecost fire fall on me
	on the day of Pentecost fire fall on me
	Pray on, pray on, pray on till Jesus come
	Pray on, pray on, pray on till Jesus come
	If your conscience set you free pray on
	Say our Father who art in heaven
	Hallowed be thy name
	Thy Kingdom come oh Lord
	Thy will be done on earth
	if your conscience set you free pray on
	When my pilot come I'll take an aeroplane ride
	I will feel so happy with Jah Jah by my side
	Sun moon and stars and it shine so bright
	when my pilot come I'll take an aeroplane ride
	Bright angel gather round me

Bright angel gather round me
Robe in white
Robe under the banner Oh
Robe in white
Robe under the banner Oh
Bright angel gather round me

Busha 1 What in the devil's name is that?
Busha 2 What in the devil's name is that?
Busha 1 I don't know old chaps
Some native ritual dance
They say, poco something
Looks more like pocomania to me
pocomania madness

All those stumblin block will have to remove
I tell you all those stumblin block will have to remove
Yes we have to break down Satan Kingdom
and build up the Church of Jah
All those stumblin block will have to remove
Modder the great stone got to move
Modder the great stone got to move
Modder the great stone, the stone of Babylon
Modder the great stone got to move
John saw them coming
John saw them coming
Coming robed in white
They all were numbered
They all were numbered
Numbered robed in white
Go before us Jah Jah go before us
go before us Jah Jah go before us
and do thy work thyself
go before Jah Jah go before us
go before Jah Jah go before us
and do thy work thyself
Roll Jordan roll, roll Jordan roll
Roll Jordan roll and do thy work thyself

Busha 1 They say it has some weird mystical powers
Busha 2 Psychic they say
Busha 1 It's related to some kind of voodoo
Busha 2 Obeah they call it
Busha 1 They say they can drive a man clean out of his mind
Busha 2 Kill him even
Carmen Come back yu nasty dutty dawg yu
come back here yu black naaga rass yu
ah wey mi baby money de
just fuck mi and gi mi pickney
go wey yu dawg yu go wey

Tek yu blood clarte out a mi muno
Ten pickney da man de breed me an lef me wid
Just mi one an Gad ina di whole blood clarte universe
    My fader is a pretty backra man wid tall pretty hair
Straight
Not like dat dutty ol naaga
Mi fix him doah de rass
Mi fix him dat de naaga man
Can't escape Princess Elizabeth
I just gather up mi parrot beak an de dawg teeth
an work a lickle nigromancy on dat black rass
Then you didn't know sey
is your worship princess you is talkin to
My fader rule over all the orbs of the universe manifest
I am a royal princess
I have my ladies in waiting who curtsey to me
My father has tall pretty hair
an him rule over all de world
An I is his princess
Uno must bow down before me, bow down
The Lord is my shepherd
I shall not want He maketh me down to lie
My fader have two white angels
with white hair and a white robe
an him rule over all de lan
an you don't joke wid my fader
you know, don't joke wid him
him wi bax yu down
like I bax down de dutty naaga man
I princess get him
cant fuck round mi an get away with it
    Ten poun ten fe go cut muno
    wai oh, wai oh
    Ten poun ten fe go cut muno
    wai oh, wai oh
    Big muno small muno fat muno
    wai oh, cut muno
    Ten poun ten fe go cut muno
    wai oh, wai oh
    Ten poun ten fe go cut muno
    wai oh, wai oh
    Red muno white muno same muno
    wai oh, cut muno
    Ten poun ten fe go cut muno
    wai oh, wai oh
    Ten poun ten fe go cut muno
    muno muno, muno muno, all the same muno

wai oh, cut muno
Mumma Mumma dem ketch puppa
dem gal dem gal from philistine
dem wine dem line like a ball of twine
If ah never run den would a ketch mi to
fe wine me line like ball of twine
When de baby come born, oh him fada
When de baby come born, oh him fada
him fada gawn a contingent
Not a sole fe sey, poor little baby
Everybody sey poor old lady

Nurse — Doctor, this man has been behaving strangely
will you look at him and tell us what you think

Doctor — Speak up man what is the problem?
Say it loud nigger, what is the problem?

Male patient — She put a duppy pon me boss
mi did promise to marry to she sar
but mi couldn't live wid har sar
she too miserable
So she set a duppy pon mi sar
She set a duppy pon mi
De duppy haig me you see sar
it haig me and haig me
So me can sleep a night time
me just tormented

Doctor — Madness, madness
what is all this talk of duppies and haig me?
what is a duppy my man?
This is madness
are all black people crazy?

Nurse — Hush doctor you have just come
It has more power than you think
Causes trouble not only amongst the blacks
But affects us too
We had to pass a law about it

Judge/Governor — On the first day of January
Which will be in the year of our Lord
One thousand seven hundred and sixty one,
Any naaga or other slave
who shall pretend any supernatural power
and be detected in making use
of any Blood, Feathers, Parrots' Beaks
Dogs' Teeth, Alligators' Teeth, Broken bottles
Grave dirt, rum, eggshells
or any other materials
related to the practice of Obeah
or witchcraft in order to delude

and impose on the minds of others
shall upon conviction thereof
before two magistrates and three freeholders
Suffer Death or Transportation.
Anything in this act or any other act
or any other law to the contrary
notwithstanding

Busha 2 But this is the year eighteen hundred and sixty one
This is one hundred years later
This is madness, it doesn't need a gallows but a madhouse
You need a madhouse a house for the mad
and we should really catch the perpetrators of this Obeah
and put an end to it

mm1 The tribe was restless
Rebellion after rebellion
We showed the Baldheads
That we wasn't goin to tek it
In 1760 Tacky almost overthrow Baldhead
and some of him own people betray him.
Pity, dem did cut off him head
and stick it pon a post near Spanish Town

mm2 Fortune and Kingston were hung in irons, alive, in Parade
Fortune lived for seven days; Kingston, nine
Testifying to the fortitude of our brave heroes

mm1 But dem dead doah

mm2 In 1831 Sam Sharpe mounted rebellion in the west

Chorus We won't lift hoe no more
we will not work no more
we won't be slaves no more
we won't take flogging no more

mm1 Don't bodder think sey dem free we cause dem love we
I man fight back an struggle an is dem have fe pay fe it

mm2 But even though Baldhead now didn't own I
Him still control I
For a him control de dunny and own all the land

Doctor I tell you my governor
What you need in the wretched colony
is a madhouse and a prison

Busha 2 Think of it in economic terms
look at all this damned trouble we are having with the niggers
The fuckers are a threat to our lives and property
Now you give them their freedom
Next thing the niggers will want to own the fucking land,
and houses and money
All you need to do is to
build a madhouse and a prison
Get the same architect to design them both, same money

then get a police force to catch them
and some warders to imprison them
and you have solved the problem
Lock all the fucking niggers away I say
I don't care whether it's madness or badness
and throw away the key

Busha 1 Of course you must employ the blacks, as warders and
constables and clerks and such the likes
We will make sure that all the officers
and medical staff and judges are all sent from the UK
but employ Blackie of course

Busha 2 In fact it is the best thing to have Blackie be his brother's jailer
Oh these black people do so love to fight with each other
Pay them a few shillings and they make the best
overseers, jailors, prison warders, what have you

Busha 1 But governor, don't show them any quarter
The only thing that Blackie really respects
is the end of a whip, or the barrel of a gun

Busha 2 Show them no mercy, mi lord show Blackie who is the boss
and he will love an respect you
Flog him within an inch of his life and he will plant your fields
cut your cane, reap your crops
and Blackie's woman will mind your children and look after your house
Show them no mercy governor, show them no mercy

Busha 1 But since this damned emancipation thing
you can't just flog the blacks just so
Wilberforce and Buxton put paid to that

Busha 2 But you can still flog him governor
Every good nigger needs a good flogging
now and again, just to keep him in order
Just make a few laws, form a police force
build a madhouse and a prison
and you can still flog him

mm1 Now I man would a like all a uno people to study
what Baldhead him did do
First him bring out a police superintendent from Englan
An jailhouse superintendent from Englan
An madhouse physician superintendent
an fi him madhouse nursing superintendent from Englan
And employ some ol naaga to put wid each of dem
if you think sey dem fuckers did mean any joke

Governor Now hear this
I want you all to realise
That in essence we are living in a time of war
Not a declared war, oh no
but an endless war with Blackie out there

to maintain an Empire
You constantly have to be on the offensive
Allow him no quarter and read him no beatitudes
The policy is very clear
divide and rule and eradicate their culture
confuse their children's heads
make suffering supreme and do not stop at torture
Go now my superintendents and do this task supreme
lock up the scum my lusty ones and we'll make quite a team
Teach them the ways of us Englishmen if you really must
but if they give you any trouble then their heads you just must bust
Remember now my loyal ones the name you carry now
Carry the flag of Empire proud
and sing the name of Queen Victoria loud

mm1 And so the madhouse was born
but I man want you all to understan
dat Babylon did see de madhouse
not as a place of treatment directly
not as a refuge
but as a jail
Babylon is just Babylon
Rasta

mm2 I man want uno fe study dem times seriously
Bellevue and Tower Street Penitentiary
did draft up at de same time

mm1 1862
Dat is de year, by fe dem calendar
dat Babylon did build de madhouse
Think of dat time
go back ina yu headcup
and get ina dem years de
Times was hard, mi brethren
Man didn't have any work either
Man didn't have no house,
I and I man did just born naked
and naked I man did live
Dem did just emancipate we
free we from slavery
dem did sey
but I man was ina
worse slavery
Dem own all de lan dem own all de factory
Dem live ina de big house
I man an I man people
did have fe find a lickle kotch here so, and dere so
ina de ghetto of the cane fields
I man don't have no learnin

dem rass hole dem wouldn't mek I go school
I man don't have no food to eat
Pickney no have no food
Dem belly a dead fe hungry
Starvation was a kill de youth dem
All kind a white man disease him bring come wid him
was just a lick down de lickle youth man dem
An you think Babylon did care
I man wasn't a human being
I man was just a animal
dat dem could just fuck around wid as dem like
Na go put up wid dat
I man want food fe eat
Want house fe sleep ina
Want clothes fe wear

Gimmie house, gimmie clothes
gimmie food fe eat
I man must hold the lan
gimmie house, gimmie clothes
gimmie food fe eat
I man must hold de lan
Yu keep all de lan an jus gi I de dregs
Yu keep all de lan an jus gi I de dregs
Gimmie house, gimmie clothes
gimmie food fe eat
I man must hold de lan

mm1 As a matter of fact Mr. Rass hole
is uno bring me ya so
so a uno must pay I fare go home
I man want to go at I yard Baldhead
Africa dat name Rasta
Sen I home to I people
an I man want to go first class
on a Concord

mm2 Dem is de time de mens build de madhouse
an de prison an de constabulary force
is dem time de me a deal wid
I and I was livin in a period of economic depression

mm1
(Paul Bogle) Paul Bogle is I name
I stan here to challenge
The authority of that ruthless white villain Governor Eyre
Downpressor of I and I people
I man demand rights and justice

Gimmie house, gimmie clothes
gimmie food fe eat
I man must hold de lan

Gimmie house, gimmie clothes
gimmie food fe eat
I man must hold de lan

mm2 Now listen Iya
I man people was demonstrating peacefully Rasta
Standin up fe dem rights an justice
When a white man name von Ketelhodt
Tell him militia man dem fe fire dem gun dem
on I an I people
Now look at dat Rasta
I an I don't have no gun
I an I don't have no bomb
an dem jus shoot we down
in cold blood

mm1 Forward I people
No bullet nah go stop I an I people
from I rights and justice
is three hundred years
we been in dis bondage
I tribe is a proud brave tribe
de man dem rise up
and kill twenty two Baldhead
wid we bare han
in de face of all dem bullet
including the boss man
Von Ketelhodt

mm2 Now di Governor man Eyre
him sey him did dreader dan dread
him sen fe him troop dem
Dem hang an shoot eighty five as dem come,
Widout any kind of trial
Dem bun down one thousan
of I an I ghetto house dem out at Morant Bay
dem flog six hundred black man and black woman
Oh gawd dat white man did wicked
Three hundred and fifty four of
I an I brethren dem court marshal
an shoot to death
just because I an I di demonstrate
for I rights an justice
an you know what dat white blood clarte
Governor man Eyre write back an tell fe him
bass dem at Englan

Governor My lords,
Retribution has been so prompt and terrible
it is never likely to be forgotten

mm2	Well you an I know how dem to white man in Englan stay
Busha 1	Oh Eyre you naughty fellow come home at once my man can't you see you are behaving like an old time slave master barbarian, my man These are modern times now, now-a-days you can't afford to treat the black people like that Think of public opinion
Busha 2	Anyhow come on home for a rest We will give you a manor and a property here and make you a lord or a baron or something
Busha 1	Thanks for your wonderful service to Empire Come and have a rest old man good show We will look after things in Jamaica
mm2	Well dem sen a next white man name Grant him was a more better white man you could even talk to him Him talk sweet you se But even through all the sweet talk him never change what him Englan bass dem did tell him fe do Uno still think sey dem did free we cause dem love we
Carmen	My fader is a tall pretty white man him pretty you see wid full straight pretty hair my fader rule over all the orbs of the universe manifest I am a royal princess I have my ladies in waiting who curtsey to me my fader has tall pretty hair an him rule over all de world an I is his princess uno must bow down before me bow down The Lord is my shepherd I shall not want he maketh me down to lie my fader have two white angels with white hair and a white robe and him rule over all de lan an yu don't joke wid my fader, you know, don't joke wid him him wi bax you down like I box down de dutty naaga man Come yah doctor come fuck me nuh fuck me
mm2	Oh yes Governor Grant got things together great reformer and liberal sweet mouth so till

you think Englan was goin to feget Bogle an Gordon dem
dem had to tek wey de old fashion wild slave master
barbarian Eyre and sen a sweet mouth

mm2
Is him write de madhouse law

Governor
Chapter one hundred and two
of the thirteenth day of August, of this year of our Lord
eighteen hundred and seventy three
Any constable may without a warrant
arrest any person whom
he shall find wandering at large
in such manner
and under such circumstances
as to devote that he is
of unsound mind
and that it would be dangerous
to continue to wander at large
and shall take him forthwith
before a
Justice of the Peace

Chorus
a Justice of the Peace?
Dread Lion ah who yu a call mad man
Dread Lion ah who yu a call mad man
Call mi man but no call me mad
Mad man
Call mi man but no call me mad
Mad man
One man cannot name mad and man
Mad man
Yu better call yu mumma so
Mad man
Yu better call yu puppa so
Mad man
Yu better call yu bredda so
Mad man
Yu better call yu sister so
Mad man
Call me man
but no call me mad
Mad man

Policeman 1
Come yah bwoy
Ah yu ah de mad man
a yu a smoke up yu ganja
an beat drum ina de night
an plot revolution and demonstration
Come yah boy
ah yu ah de man man
yu must be name

	Communist
mm2	Communist?
	Ah wey you find dat name
	Ah mad man him name
mm2	Call I Jah Rastafari
	Dreadie
Policeman 1	Mi no care who de rass yu is, yu is a fuckin mad man
	an I an I ah go lock yu up ina de jail house
	and den sen yu to the madhouse
mm1	Sen who?
	Sen yu mumma
	Sen yu puppa
	What I man do
	leggo leggo
	cause I man eating calliweed
	Sen mi go wey
	a madhouse
	yu mad to rass
	no lock I up
	go wey an leave I man alone
Policeman 1	What?
	Dis ya mad man ah resist arrest from de arresting Constable
	grab him men, grab him ina him waist
	burst him head wide open
	Then tie him up in a special ganzy
	made of canvas tied behind
	with a special design
	you'll look pretty in this chemise
	designed to give you plenty breeze
	but movements not a squeeze
Judge	Any Justice of the Peace
	upon information being laid
	before him by oath
	that any person within the courts
	of his jurisdiction has been, or is
	wandering at large
	and is deemed to be of unsound mind
	and that it will be dangerous
	to permit such a person
	to continue to wander at large
	or that it would be better
	for such a person
	that he should be detained in the Mental Hospital
	and bring him before any Justice of the Peace
	What did he do?
Policeman 1	Set a fire to four cane fields mi Lud
Judge	He must be mad

When he destroys those canes
he reduces the amount of work for
himself and his family
Say what?
He smokes ganja
Constable

Policeman 1 He is one of those ganja smokers
How often yu smoke boy?

Judge Spit in my face you black dirty, dirty
you will pay for this nigger
That man is a mad man
he will be incarcerated in the Mental Hospital
for the rest of his natural life
Just tell those two doctors to fill out the certificates
Tell them the story that he has a violent tendency this one
He will murder and steal
furthermore he expresses great hostility to white people
This makes him doubly dangerous
Tell doctor to be especially careful with this one
when you get him to the Lunatic Asylum
he is a mad black buck

mm2 But a who dem people deh eh?
a wey dem come from?
But a dem de ah de true Babylon
the Constable, the Justice of the Peace
the Lunatic Asylum
ah who mad ah you?
Ah dat said Grant
de one wid de sweet mout ah him cause it
you think sey dem free yu because dem love you
you think dat because him laugh and talk sweet wid you
him is any different from the one Eyre

mm1 All white people look
alike

Governor Law Eight, April 1st, Eighteen hundred and sixty seven
Organization of Semi-military Constabulary Force
As Governor of this Colony I pass this law
To replace the old Police Force
in consequence of the inefficiency of the old police of the island
This inefficiency had been demonstrated by
the evils of 1865
The men are enlisted for five years
and before they are posted in the several parishes
they undergo military training
as well as civil instruction
at a central depot in Spanish Town
established in the Old Military Barracks

When on ordinary duty they carry batons
but when ordered out under arms
being under military organization
They would be able to overawe to instantly to repress
even such a violent and lawless demonstration as occurred in 1865

mm2 Don't bodder think sey dem free yu
because dem love yu

Busha 1 Grant got the Colony settled though
Good man Grant
knows how to deal with niggers
Especially niggers these days

Jane and Louisa will soon come home
will soon come home, will soon come home
Jane and Louisa will soon come home
into this beautiful garden
My love will you allow me to pluck a rose
yes to pluck a rose yes to pluck a rose
my love will you allow me to pluck a rose
into this beautiful garden
Jane and Louisa will soon come home
will soon come home, will soon come home
Jane and Louisa will soon come home
into this beautiful garden

Governor Nothing like a little good music to soothe the brow
and one thing you can say for Blackie
he certainly knows how to make music

Busha 1 Gifted that way black people
oh yea
gifted that way

Busha 2 Had to take away their drums from them after 1865
Causing too much trouble with Blackie on the plantation

Busha 1 Strange things, those drums
These people use them to communicate with each other

Busha 2 Had to ban them after sixty five
too dangerous

Governor Now let them play quadrille
Keep down their pressure good clean healthy fun
when they are finished on the plantation
In fact I think I'll teach them cricket too
Jane and Louisa will soon come home
into this beautiful garden
Now hear this

SMO As physician superintendent and Senior Medical Officer
of this Lunatic Asylum
I have one responsibility keep those mad men
off the streets
one thing I do not allow in this Asylum

is for any of the inmates to escape
Matron
when you recruit staff for this institution
I want big strapping black men and women
To work as warders
If any of you allow any of them to escape
you will be out on the street
with no job
Hear me clear
you will give me a muster of all the inmates
Morning and evening
Report every absconder
And the warder who let him escape
will surely lose the work
One meal per day is all they'll get
and lock them down all day and night
Nobody want to visit a mad man
but if any relatives want to visit they can come
Remember
mad people have no rights
The lunatics who come here
come for the rest of their lives
So just find a secure corner and lock them far away
And don't be afraid to bust his head
if he gives you any trouble
Those that don't give trouble
let them get some exercise
but make sure they can't go further
Than you can see them
They are not to be trusted even then
They might just kill you
yes even that
And when the SMO or the Matron come around
jump to attention; salute, and say
'all correct and reported for Sir'.
An if you make any of these mad people escape
you will face severe disciplinary action
and you will lose your job immediately

Male attendant — Man have to mek a living somehow
but we did have to look out for dem
because dem is we bredda

mm1 — Fights between inmates were the order of the day
Overcrowding, and serious conditions of filth
and human degradation
Attendants were hand picked
they had to be big hefty men to control those patients
Fights were the order of the day

mm2	Bust dem head yes 'Mist punches' treatment prescribed by our colonial doctor 'Mist punches' was on the treatment ticket we had to defend weself when a fe we life de pon de wicket
Male attendant	Of course it was illegal to beat a patient but a man have a right to defend himself an after all whitey pay I money to mek sure dat the inmate dem don't escape
mm2	Arrest that mad man, lock him up tie him with fetters bold keep him locked in hospital until he is quite old
mm1	Seclusion was the order of the day The doctor's orders were that patients should be locked away for twelve hours of each day with an hour for lunch in between
Female attendant	I am an attendant and let me tell you the life was grim I had to work for whitey and him didn't treat we much different From de lunatic dem
Male attendant	Make sure that the patients didn't get away For the Busha doctor man don't play If a patient get wey you suffer then you know sey dawg nyam you supper
mm1	Dat is I Senior Medical Officer but me no know how come he did call him 'Medical' Dat man de was more like a jailer
mm2	Dem did have one SMO dat did walk up an down the Asylum at night time wid him gun You hear what mi sey One of dem long mout shot gun, an shoot after anything dat move ina de night time darkness
mm1	So don't mek you feel sey dem bring I here fe treat I dem bring I here fe control I because dem can't manage I an I out deh ha ha ha ha So dem did bring I here an lock I up I man sey dat nothing didn't do me
Bedward	My name is Alexander Bedward I am destined to die in this madhouse for twenty seven years I have nurtured and tended to my flock like the good shepherd in the pasture but because dem lock me in de madhouse

dey think that they can keep me from my people
Dem white people been after I Alexander Bedward for forty years
Way back in eighteen ninety four, dem arrest I an lock I up for sedition
Brothers an sisters some thirty years have passed
since our brothers Bogle and Gordon were hanged
along with our heroic brethren of the time
who rose up against that barbarian Eyre
My brothers and sisters how long must we remain in bondage?
Enslave us for three hundred years and then emancipate us into bondage
Brothers and sisters we are still living in that slavery
Oh yes but now dem dress it up
yu think anything change since 1830, since 1865?
This is the year of our lord eighteen hundred and ninety four
an times don't change
brothers and sisters we still under bondage same way
Ah fe we brethren dem dat dem shoot down in cold blood in 1865
Morant Bay
don't forget Bogle, brothers
don't forget Gordon, sisters
Look around you brothers and sisters
who lives in the big house, who has the grand carriage, who owns the land
It is the big man, the white man
Babylon
Black people, black people why can't we ever learn
these white people mean us every harm?
Hypocrites, hypocrites, robbers, thieves
they laugh and joke and smile with you
discuss the time of day
but misery for black people still don't change
and we still have fe wuk pon backra massa lan
Hypocrites, hypocrites, robbers, thieves

Governor
Arrest dat man and lock him down
He is disturbing the peace
He is dangerous
He is seditious
He is bad he is mad
Arrest that man and lock him down
he has altogether too much to say
and too much sway over the people

Lawyer 1
Mi Lud
I put it to you that Mr. Bedward
was deliberately and seditiously inciting
the people into rebellion against the crown
Inciting the people into civil disobedience, mi Lud

he is bad and must be mad
He also runs a Church mi Lud
and claims that the Hope River has some healing powers.
Practices baptismal healing and balm yard cures
he is altogether a dangerous fellow
we have had a number of complaints
send him to the Lunatic Asylum
Yes mi Lud

Sly mongoose yuh name gawn abroad
Sly mongoose yuh name gawn abroad
Mongoose go in a Bedward Kitchen
tek out one of him righteous chicken
put it ina him waistcoat pocket
Sly mongoose
Sly mongoose yuh name gawn abroad
Sly mongoose yuh name gawn abroad

Lawyer 2 Mi Lud
I appear on behalf of my client Alexander Bedward
who has been declared a lunatic
and committed to the Lunatic Asylum
With respect mi Lud
this seems to be a totally inappropriate and unjust punishment
to a man who has committed no crime
more than preaching the word of his God to his people

Judge Appeal upheld
Release Alexander Bedward

Dip dem Bedward, dip dem
Dip dem in de healing stream
Dip dem Bedward
Dip dem in de healing stream
Dip dem Bedward, dip dem
Dip dem fe cure bad feeling
Dip dem Bedward, dip dem
Dip dem in de healing stream
Dip dem Bedward, dip dem
Dip dem fe cure bad feeling

Bedward Behold Brethren the Lamb of God who is come amongst you
to preach the doctrine of the black man's God
To preach the power of the black man's soul
To teach redemption from sin
of the avoidance of evil
of the power of faith
of the glory of love
of the cleansing discipline of fasting
and the purifying faith of Baptism
Shun hypocrisy and deceit
and believe that the strength and power of the

black man can make him move mountains
can make him fly
Fly to Zion with me to Zion
and deliverance from Babylon.
Sly mongoose yuh name gawn abroad
Sly mongoose yuh name gawn abroad
Mongoose go in a Bedward kitchen
tek out one of him righteous chicken
put it ina him waistcoat pocket
Sly mongoose
Sly mongoose yuh name gawn abroad
Sly mongoose yuh name gawn abroad
Dip dem Bedward, dip dem
dip dem in de healing stream
Dip dem Bedward, dip dem
dip fe cure bad feeling

mm1 For twenty seven years Bedward preached his gospel
For twenty seven years Bedward dodged Baldhead
Baldhead try every trick to lock him up but him pop dem
Finally dem see him back to madhouse
sey him mad cause him mobilise thousands of black people
to rekindle their burning desire to return to Zion

mm2 White man sey him mad
Seh him a tell people
Fe fly off a tree to heaven
what a thing.
Bedward dead in a my hand dem
dem did try fe downpress fe him spirit
but dat old man beam out goodness and love
till the day him dead
Babylon man did sey him mad
and mek up story bout him
fui.
Feel sey I wanna be free
feel sey I wanna be free
I have so many questions
Feel sey I wanna be free
Feel sey I wanna be free
What about my human rights?
I wanna be free
I feel sey I wanna be free

ACT II

mm2 *Step by step we goin to the golden gate*
Step by step we goin to the gate
Wey de righteous must stan an de wicked must fall
Only the pure will answer to the call
Wey de righteous must stand an de wicked must fall
Only the pure will answer to the call

Step by step we goin to the golden gate
Step by step we goin to the gate
Wey de wicked dem a drop and de humble de pon top
de road is long as we leave Babylon
Wey de wicked dem a drop and de humble de pon top
de road is long and we leave Babylon
Step by step we goin to the golden gate
Step by step we goin to the gate
When me reach Zion
the victory will be grand
Only Jah man will stan up in that land

mm3 Hey
Come yah
mister gentleman
You want a pair of shoes
to buy
I man have
a nice pair of brown loafers
to sell de man

Gentleman Shoes
Mi no want to buy no shoes from no madman
next ting you know is two left foot
you can't trust you Bellevue people
You known

mm3 No boss, no
me is a poor unfortunate man
bass
I man don't have no fader and madder
and den some police did come an invade
I home an bruck down I door and lock I up
and sen I here to Bellevue sar
I is a poor man sar
Mi ah go sell you de shoes cheap sar
Cheap cheap
Only fifteen shillin sar
Fifteen shillin fi dis ya boots sar
You can't want a better shoes
or a better bargain sar
patronise a poor Bellevue madman sar
only fifteen shillin sar
Coo de quality of de boot

Gentleman Hm Hm! dem really look pretty fe tru
Is wey you get dis pretty
shoes from boy
You must be thief dem
eh boy

mm3 No bass No

	Ah bran new shoes Mi wife did sen for me from 'Merica sar But dem can't fit me bass, dem just can't fit me But dem wi fit you bass, dem wi fit you
Gentleman	How much you sey you want fi dem? Fifteen shillings You must be crazy boy fifteen shilling in dis ya hard time I would be a mad man fe buy dem shoes at dat price
mm3	Lawd backra you know sey fifteen shillin fe dem ya shoe is a bargain sar is ten pound fe dem on Kings Street don't vantage me sar because I poor Fifteen shillin a bargain bass, a bargain
Gentleman	You mus be think sey me is de mad man fifteen shillin fe dat shoes Mi wi give you ten shillin tek it or leave it
mm3	Ten shillin bass, Oh gawd bass is a sin, is a sin beg mercy no bass, beg mercy I is a poor man is only fifteen shillin mi ask you bass
Gentleman	Mi sey mi will give you ten shillin fe it tek it or leave it
mm3	All right sar, all right, mi we tek it, but is a sin, sar, is a sin
Gentleman	All right dem give mi de shoes them
mm3	You have to give me my money first sar I am a Bellevue madman sar, but mi no fool sar me no fool
Gentleman	All right You too damn facety, Hey, see your money dey Now give me de shoes
mm3	Yes sar see it here sar, try on dis ya foot see how it look pon you try it on sar
Gentleman	Bwoy, what a way the boot boasy bredda Ah 'Merican boot dis you know Come, gimmie de next foot madboy, gimmie de next foot
mm3	Is ten pound fe de odder foot sar

Gentleman	You mad Don't mi just pay you mi ten shillin just gimmie de odder shoes and walk off mad man
mm3	No sar Ah you must walk off is ten shillin fe dat foot of shoes an ten poun fe dis foot you can tek it or leave it
Gentleman	You dam ginal you how come you so smart an you ina Bellevue gimmie de odder foot of shoes mad man
mm3	Ten pound or no shoes sar
Gentleman	Ah me must be de mad man lawd de boot pretty fe true Mi can afford fe lose dis yah 'Merican boot All right, all right see de ten pound here now gimmie de shoes mad boy
mm3	Oh yes sar, wid pleasure sar see de shoes here so sar
Gentleman	Dam theifing Bellevue mad man Gimmie de shoes Lawd de shoes pretty sar pretty fe true You can see I when I step out wid I beef tonight But wait how come dis ya foot of shoes can't go pon mi foot Wait, wait, is two left foot You know is two left foot shoes dat mad man sell me Hey you theifing mad rass you Gimmie back me money, gimmie back me money me ah go bring police fe arrest you you theifing ginal you, gimmie back me money Mek ah ever catch you I stone out you clothes and bust you mout Me a go fe de police fe arrest you rass go-wey mad man
mm3	Who de cap fits let him wear it Mi think sey him was only going to throw back one foot of de shoes dem Him lucky ah shoulda did charge him twelve poun ten fe de shoe dem Hey come ya Mister gentleman You want a pair of shoes to buy I man have a nice pair of brown loafers to sell de man
mm1	Is so my brethren stay You must excuse him

	it makes you wonder though about who should be here and who should be there But when you live in a place like Bellevue You soon learn how to live Look ya man ina dis yah place You spen every day of yu life lock up behind iron bars wid nothing to do but plait sand and stone breeze
mm2	You ever hear of two hundred mad man, lock up together in a de same room, eating together, sleeping together playing together, fighting together what a crosses an nobody really care dem have fe live so year after year
mm1	De first thing a man want to do When dem bring him some a Bellevue is to escape, run wey.
Policeman 1	Is you is de admitting nurse mam? Me bring a man fe admit a Bellevue Him mad you see mam it tek six a we fe hold him down
Policeman 2	But we arrest him an tie him up in a special ganzy made of canvas and tied behind designed to give him plenty breeze but movements not a squeeze
Nurse	No Mister Constable, you nah lef him yeh tie up like any chicken in a you special ganzy you know sey dat me have to receive a patient not a man ina straight jacket
Policeman 1	Den loose him off den nuh loose off de cord dem and roll him out
Policeman 2	Wait, don't mek him get wey come back boy come back yah
Male nurse 1	Same thing now what uno policeman know bout mad man come back here boy an if you give me any trouble ah goin to bust you mouth
Male nurse 2	See it yah pon your treatment ticket de doctor write sey I must give you 'mist punches' if you feget yuself
Male nurse 1	You know is what dat it mean sey a thump ina you mout an a big lick ina you back
Male nurse 2	Ah fe you doctor write up dat de treatment fe you boy, so learn dat Now go ina da cell yah and shet up yu mout mi don't want no noise ina de ward tonight

I come yah fe sleep tonight
Mi have work fe do tomorrow up a Nuttall,
is mi day off
mm1 Life of de black man did hard
But de life of de mad black man harder still
is nuff nuff punishment I man been under from Babylon land
an it bitter me a tell you, bitter
You see Bedward him mek one mistake
Him call himself Jesus Christ
and de white man lock him up
sey him a mad man.
Consider dat mi brethren
Jesus Christ did sey him was the son of God
Born of the Virgin Mary
conceive of de Holy Ghost
Now, a whole heap of people believe dat
around de world till now
Den what
dis black man come on yah
him sey dat him is de son of God, de black man God
an a whole heap of people believe dat
around dis yah lan till now
An him did mobilize de people dem from cross de lan St. Elizabeth,
Westmoreland man come from far an wide to follow dat man
But him mek one mistake
him not only tell de white man dat he is the son of God
but dat him is Jesus Christ
dem couldn't tek dat, dem arrest him
Say him a mad man an throw him ina de Asylum
mm2 But Marcus Garvey him never mek de same mistake
Babylon nuh try fe lock Marcus down nuff time but dem fail
an him never mek the same mistake
As the Jew is held together by his religion
The white races by the assumption and the rule of superiority
and the Mongolian by the special tie of blood
So likewise the negro must be united in one great racial hierarchy
Negroes the world over must practice one faith
That of confidence in our enlightenment
'With One God, One Aim, One Destiny
Let sky and God be our limit and Eternity our measurement
Let no voice but your own speak to you from the depths
Let no influence but your own arouse you in time of peace and time of war'
mm1 Oh so you know wey we reach we de ina de nineteen thirties
the time of all kind of bangarang ina de world
Bedward did just dead,
Marcus Garvey was a confuse up de American white man head

Hitler was a rise in Europe de Fascist vanguard
An Selassie was a fight Mussolini back a yard
The world capitalist system was taking a beating
at the time of the crash when Wall Street did mash
Ghandi was walking the streets of Bombay
and Ho Chi Minh fought the French in his own heroic way
Mao Tse Tung did start fe him long march
And Stalin the Dread was helping Siberia get ahead
mm2 While back home on the ranch things did a hot up outa street
St. William Grant and Bustamante up an down the country
Coombs, Buchanan and Norman Manley in de streets
The working class movement was just ah born
The people was a rise up against backra massa
White man rule was a bruck
Gimmie house, gimmie clothes, gimmie good fe eat
I man ah go strike, mi nah wuk
mm3 You nuh understan wey I man mean
No goods or clothes for King street, seen
Me a go lock down the dock
Bruck chain and padlock
Me nah cut no more sugar cane
Shillin an hour was the strikers claim
mm1 The working class movement was born
for one hundred years backra massa wouldn't allow
I man working class to form one union
Well in de thirties de union dem did draft up an fight
and start agitate fe for black working people right
Dem was a fight down the colonial oppressors of I and I
The colonial government that did control from Whitehall
the colonial owners of land, plantation and business freight
Ah dem I and I working people rise up an challenge in '38
mm2 Is a funny thing
De same English white man dem who did flog me
downpress abuse and torture we
lock me up fe smoke calli weed
Shoot me down in the streets in cold blood
When I an I a demonstrate fi I rights an justice an work
Ah de same English white government who did
a fight down Hitler because him did want fi rule dem
mm1 You see it dey
anader white Garman man want to rule Mrs. Queen and Mr. King
who a rule over I and I black man still
mm2 An Mr. King a fight down Hitler because Adolph an him Fascist clan
Treat de Jews like how backra massa treat us enslaved African
fe four hundred years
mm1 Hypocrites, hypocrites, liars, thieves
The white race is the cruellest, most sadistic of the races of fealty

Wars an instruments of wars have been their specialty
They created capitalism the economic system
Used to downpress I freedom exploit I labour and grow fat from I sufferin
An is dem now a mek all de gun and de boom dem
mm2 In 1938 I people rose up to show Babylon
that me put up wid sufferin and deprivation for four hundred years
an I man was a get vex because mi did tell yu say long time ago
fi let me go, let me go, an leave I and man alone
Gimmie back mi shillin wid de lion pon it
wid de lion pon it wid de lion pon it
Gimmie back mi shillin wid de lion pon it
Gal you must be tek me fe a fool
Not because you so big an fat
gal you must think sey me fraid fe dat
gal you must be tek me fe a fool
Mi drink white rum till me tumble dung
mi no want dutty gal come fingle me
Oh de woman ina kitchen she a grumble sey she want go home
Oh de woman ina kitchen she a grumble sey she want go home
Cookie pick up de fine she put on de cinnamon tea pon fire
Oh de woman ina kitchen she ketch up de fire
she put on de cinnamon tea pon fire
Oh de woman in a kitchen she a grumble sey she want go home
mm1 Inside a dis yah madhouse
things couldn't be worse
Boil yam ina de skin[1] gi mi
lock me up in a pit latrine
don't gimmie nuff food fe eat
I want to go home a mi yard
I am the Virgin Mary, Mother of God
Want to go home a mi yard
listen nuh darlin
dem sey him a batty man
dat man sar dat man
oh him ah beat me sar
Just leave mi things alone
mek a thump you ina yu mout
Patient Want food fe eat, want man
Nurse I want more food fe eat
Nurse I want more food fe eat
Nurse tek me off a de canvas bed no, do
beg yu tek me off ah de canvas bed nurse do

[1]To '*boil yam in the skin*' is a practice reserved for the preparation of food for pigs, and reflects an insult showing the utmost disrespect.

mi can't sleep pon de concrete floor
Nurse, beg yu a cigarette
gimmie a quattie nuh, gimmie a quattie

Carmen
I am the Virgin Mary, Mother of God
too much crab louse an chink ina I bed Sister
Mi can't sleep a night time wid de bitin an de scratchin everlastin
Hey a mi chop up de maga man de
cut him ina him tripe
mi wi chop you up too
Nurse, mi want lickle water
gimmie lickle crackers fe eat nuh
Nurse me wi throw de dede
all over yu uniform
I am Virgin Mary, Mother of God
Too much crab louse ina dis ya place
Nurse, mi wi cut yu ina yu tripe
Jesus Christ my Lord and saviour
is long time now me want fe chop up a nurse
I am the Virgin Mary, Mother of God
Mi did tell you sey dat if you did
touch mi things me was goin thump yu

Patient
Thump me an mi a go thump you back
Ha ha ha ha
ha ha
ha ha
ha ha ha ha

Nurse
Lord Jesus Johnny mi can't stan dis yah place
You know mi can't stan dis ya madhouse
is three years now mi come to work at dis ya
madhouse as a nurse an mi can't tek it no more

Male nurse 1
All right Maisie, take it easy
tell me what happened today
I never see you stay so before
what happen to you

Nurse
Is dis ya madhouse Johnny I can't tek it
You know what the kitchen sen down today
Yam boil ina de skin
Yu hear mi
Not even pig could a eat dat de sinting
an is dat we have fe eat is a sin an a disgrace

mm1
Is true, an inside dat de B ward,
it have so much chink and bed bug
me no know how dem don't
nyam off de patient dem

Nurse
Lock down de madhouse
Lock it down
me nah wuk no more

till the workers have justice an rights
freedom from colonial downpression
freedom from Babylon

mm1 For three weeks the nurses picketed the hospital
they closed the gates it was a very heroic act
because they were the first group of workers to go
on strike for improved conditions for themselves and the patients
and not only for better wages

mm2 For three weeks Bellevue Hospital was run
by volunteers, dock workers and the army

mm1 They call that strike Black Saturday
and it occurred in 1946
That was the birth of the working class
movement in Bellevue Hospital
The brave nurses who defied backra massa for three weeks
Were severely punished
Many were not rehired, others lost their pension rights
and all other privileges

Nurse It was there at the picket line we realized that the only way
to achieve our rights was for the workers to struggle

Nurse 2 Rise up the working class
Unite black people
take the power from backra massa
and do thy work thyself

mm1 The inmates of Bellevue had a ball while the strike raged
and the struggle was waged
I man bredda inside of Bellevue celebrated
Man run free and burn down the sports pavilion
Happy days were here again

mm1 But a what do dem mi no know
what dem mad man ah jump up an down so fa

mm2 Dem happy
because dem come
together an fight
an struggle

Carmen An we win de prize

mm1 Win which prize?
ah which prize yu think sey yu win?
Yu think sey yu a go win prize ina dem white people sinting
Just because sey uno mad man can get wey an jump up an down
an don't have nobady fe guard house uno?
No think sey is so out dey really stay

mm2 It dread out dey Rasta
Dread out de

mm1 Yes all right the workers of Bellevue fight an struggle
an show backra massa sey dat dem was
ah treat we an de patient dem worse dan any animal

mm1 So you sey dat because de white man dem sen
Cameron an fe him matron home to Englan
dat de struggle did over
what
the battle did just start
mm2 Dem Englan man dem smart yu know yu fegat sey is fe
four hundred years him did control Empire
mm1 Well look here now what him do
Him sen wey Cameron and mek a Jamaican docta as boss
him gi de workers dem some a de dregs
mm2 True things was little better but is jus de dregs
for dem couldn't treat fe dem mad people
an fe dem workers in Englan de same way
mm1 So dem gi we de dregs wid dem sweet mouth
an dem split up de working people
an put de Jamaican backra massa fe rule we
Instead, after all dat struggle an fighting
we find weself widout pension rights
some a we lose de work an black men still a fight amongst themselves
dem call it Universal Adult Suffrage but ah Universal Capitalistic Suffrage
mm2 Yu better believe sey is just anodor way
fe divide dem and rule we
black man him so ignorant him just love fe fight down
him bredda fe de last lickle thing
mm1 By the early fifties working class people were hopelessly divided
an fighting wid each other everybody a migrate to Englan
You remember when people sell dem cow,
dem goat, dem donkey just fe go a de lan
wey milk and honey flow and gold line de street
what a thing
mm2 An yu know is dat white racist Enoch Powell
invite black people fe go ah Englan fe look work ina de fifties
him was Minister of Health in Englan den
Now him a run we, sey we fe go ah we yard
mm1 When cold bite I brethren ina de white man lan
an him see fe himself how de white man stay in fe him own lan
an dat de only gold dat line de streets ina Englan
mek from de blood of I an I black people
An den things in Bellevue didn't change too much
whole heap ah Bellevue workers did go a foreign too
In ah Bellevue dem did stop beat de patient dem so much
but electro convulsive therapy an sodium amytal ina yu batty
can hurt you worse dan a thump ina yu mout
mm2 The structure, de law dem, de backra massa mentality
dat never change an black man still
don't have no food no clothes, no work

an dem still a lock up man fe smoke calli weed
an de working class did split up
Gentleman But wait
me never know say dem did mek madman walk wid cutlass
den suppose sey him jus, him jus
Hello nice Mr. Bellevue man
Hello sir, nice man from Bellevue
But ah wonder why dis ya Bellevue madman
jus a stan up ah look pan mi wid him lass ina him han
But see yah everywhere mi go dis mad man a go deh
See ya if me walk slow dis ya mad man walk slow back ah mi
if me walk fast him walk fast too wid de lass ina him han
Lawd Jesas beg yu sah, do sah
Lawd Jesas do sah do
me is de only son mi mumma have sah
do sah, do sah
Our Fader, which art in heaven
hallowed be thy name,
Lawd mi done now
mi ded now
See mi here Fader
mm3 One two three last lick
is your turn fi catch mi now
come nuh
Ah penny wheel oh a penny wheel
wheel wheel wheelie wheel oh
Wey mek yu push yu cushy gi mi penny wheel
Wey mek yu push yu cushy gi mi penny wheel
An a rub out mu muno penny wheel
a penny wheel
Ah penny wheel oh a penny wheel
wheel wheel wheelie wheel oh
Male nurse 1 Strike, strike, workers strike
mm1 Dem time we ina de late nineteen fifties
tings dem did well dread ina dis yah lan
an all over de world
people worldwide decide sey dem nah tek
no more punishment an decide fe go fight down
backra massa once an for all
mm2 Right next door ah we Fidel Castro an de great Che
was a throw out backra massa ina de fem lan Cuba
dem did come pon de *Granma* an fight Batista ina de Sierra Maestra
an de white man dem did try fe sey dat Fidel
was a mad man what a thing
Fidel win dem doah, him run out US
imperialist forces out a fe him lan
an free fe him people dem

	an dat did ah go on right next door to we in Jamaica
	an fe we backra massa
	did frighten an try fe hold back dat news
	from I an I people
mm1	An US imperialism, self-proclaimed protector of freedom around de globe
	start fe fight down poor people around de world
	Guatemala, South America, Africa, de America white man
	find himself wid him money an him gun an bomb dem
	an downpress de poor people around de world
mm2	Him did think sey dat because it was poor people
	black people, yellow people him coulda jus walk in
	an beat dem down like him beat down de
	black people dem ina fe him back yard, in Georgia
	South Carolina, Mississippi
	but Fidel stop him, Ho Chin Minh in Viet Nam
	fight him down an dem run out Yankee
	imperialism outa fe dem lan
	An de same thing was a happen right here in Jamaica
mm1	De same time Fidel was a fight down Batista
	ina de Sierra Maestra Mountain
	Rastafari was a rise up ina fe we Blue Mountains
	Claudius Henry an fi him brethren dem was a fight down
	white man rule ina Clarendon, St. Catherine
	an did mount rebellion ina Coral Gardens in Montego Bay
mm2	An right here ina Bellevue Don Drummond was a
	tell we bout Eastern Standard Time
Group circle	Mek we hold a pipe an go ina we headcup
	Me have a pipe right here so
	Lock all crowns
mm1	Man mek pipe outa bockle Rasta, a just so
	Cant tek wey I drew Rasta, even out ya so de pon de stage
	so even though dem lock I up Rasta I man just a go de
mm3	Yu can get de best ganja ina de prison and de madhouse
mm2	I remember sey Don was a tell I sey dat we a live ina fe dem time
	an we a still slave fe Babylon ina fe him time
mm1	You know sey da in Africa
	Thousands of years ago
	some of I brethren develop fe we own calendar
	four days ina de seek, seven week a month
	an de month run wid de moon
	Rastafari
mm2	Eastern Standard Time
	a dat the Don did a tell I
mm3	Lock all crowns
	give thanks an praise
	to the most high

Jah Rastafari
mm1 But Babylon did a tell
I sey thirty days
have September, April
June and November
all the rest have
Thirty one, except
February dat ah
de bastard pickney
dat ah fe dem calendar
an fe four hundred year dem condition
I an I brain sey a so it go
mm2 Come out da dirts Rasta
dem deh a Sodom an Gomorra
come outa Babylon go ina yu headcup
an beat down dat dirts
mm1 By de way
is not really ganja I man have ina
dis bockle
dem have some crazy laws about ganja smoking
So I man can't smoke ganja pon de stage
Yu think sey is we who is schizophrenic in yah
Go wey, ah yu
mm2 Mi no sey I mad Rasta,
but yu listen to I an I reasoning
if yu tell a man sey dat de world did flat Rasta
don't him wi tell you sey you mad
mm3 But Rasta
don't is just bout five hundred
years ago, all white man
dem did think sey de world flat Rasta
mm1 An him was a beat down
I an I man when I tell him sey dat a foolishness
dat I man did penetrate around de whole world
thousands of years before ina canoe
mm2 Yu never see a thing like dat Rasta
Ah de same white man
who was a lock I up ina chain
I up to build up fe him Empire
an call I inferior
an a secon class animal because I black
ah de said white man ah fight man down
when I tell him sey dat de world round
Everything dat de white man a tell you Iyia
a come out a fe him headcup
an a fe him experience an den him sey
dat because you don't think like him dat you is backward

The white man a mek all de folly ina de world
den a who backward
de man who fight an love fe kill him bredda
mm1 The white races have murdered
more than one hundred million
black people in de past four hundred years
mm1 Dat did work out at two hundred an fifty thousan every year Rasta
An dem still a shoot dem down now Rasta
Soweto, Angola, Zimbabwe, Namibia
South Africa, South Carolina, Mississippi
mm2 Bellevue in the seventies was in turmoil
strike after strike I an I black people waged
struggling for better conditions for us the working people
and I an I patients
We run out the Jamaican SMO early ina de seventies
cause backra massa rule no change
mm1 Then Michael Manley start to tell the people dem
bout democratic socialism an Munroe him talk bout full socialism
An Jah people was a ask what dis thing really mean
an dem start fi go ina dem headcup
mm2 And in Bellevue the struggle intensified
an now some a de nurse dem
a fight down de Doctor Dread Eskimo
because him cuss too much bad wud
an wear open-toe slippers
But all dat nah go fool I an I working people
we know where we ah go an what we are doing
for we know sey what we a go on wid now
is just no show
that we know what we are doing
and where we ah go
Gimmie house, gimmie clothes
gimmie food fe eat
I man must hold de lan
mm1 Now hear this brothers and sisters
we must rebuild our society for the successful
Iration of I situation
scientifically, irecally
under the guidance of
Jah Jah workers
Rastafari,
No man must own for private gain
Vank Babylon again and again
lock exploitation of man by man
and order productivity for I hand
mm2 Babylon cannot remain
the bastion of power

we must dismantle that domain
and let Jah working people reign
Take all power from Babylon
and establish the power of Jah man
together workers all must rule
and to learn this we must go to school
Special mention I man must make
of the difference which does prevail
of man who work and live Jah plan
Together we will walk hand in hand
step by step, and the victory will be grand
when no man will own a piece of sand
and set I free in Zion land
mm1 Jah farmer and his queen
the higglers from Papine
The doctors, lawyers, teachers too
will join to make a team
Beat down Babylon an fi him team
don't mek we lose the guiding beam
Jah workers must control the land
and write the lines of Zion plan
mm2 Release I an I man culture
For all to see, to love, to be
give all man work in this ya land
then find you centre, plan carefully
Those who were second before
become those who dictate the terms
creating the culture of I and I
give thanks and praise, Jah Rastafari
How do we know that this is so
Just look around, watch Babylon go
as the workers of Mount Zion I unite
Babylon quails and love prevails
For there is no work in Babylon
and pickney starving still
the big man him a mek more and more
and capital still is king
mm2 But crisis after crisis Babylon does face
where money has no value
many workers lose their jobs
as imperialism giggles
Poor people of the world have called
for their economic right
Vank capitalism they declare
and give me what is mine

Step by step we goin to the golden gate
Step by step we goin to the gate

Wey de righteous must stan an de wicked must fall
Only the pure will answer to the call
Wey de righteous must stan an de wicked must fall
Only the pure will answer to the calll
Step by step we goin up to Zion Land
Step by step we goin up to Zion Land
Wey de wicked dem a drop and de humble de pon top
de road is long as we leave Babylon
Wey de wicked dem a drop and de humble de pon top
de road is long as we leave Babylon
Step by step we goin to the promised land
Step by step we goin to the promised land
When me reach Zion the victory will be grand
Only Jah man will stan up in that land

mm1 So you see why de madhouse now
we ah change up the place
an dem a fight we
Nothing naw go stop I and I people
we just ah go change the madhouse Iyia
an come out of here
We thank you for taking time out
to visit our madhouse frolic
come back an see dem show
again an again
remember we nah jester bout dis
Rasta, so when you go out side
open yu headcup wide
an step into the land of the free
an remember sey
is Trummie tell you dat

Index

F. W. Hickling, *Decolonization of Psychiatry in Jamaica*,
https://doi.org/10.1007/978-3-030-48489-7

N

O

The manufacturer's authorised representative in the EU is Springer Nature Customer Service Centre GmbH, Europaplatz 3, 69115 Heidelberg, Germany. If you have any concerns regarding our products, please contact ProductSafety@springernature.com

Printed and bound by CPI Group (UK) Ltd, Croydon, CR0 4YY
22/09/2026
02220948-0002